Note

Healthcare practice and knowledge are constantly changing and developing as new research and treatments, changes in procedures, drugs and equipment become available.

The editors and publishers have, as far as is possible, taken care to confirm that the information complies with the latest standards of practice and legislation.

Younger mothers and older mothers:
Maternal age and maternity care

Edited by

Tracey A Mills, Debbie M Smith and Dame Tina Lavender

QUAY BOOKS
A division of MA Healthcare Ltd

Quay Books Division, MA Healthcare Ltd, St Jude's Church, Dulwich Road, London SE24 0PB

British Library Cataloguing-in-Publication Data
A catalogue record is available for this book

ISBN-10: 1-85642-438-3
ISBN-13: 978-1-85642-438-7

Edited by Jessica Anderson

Cover design by Bexi Harris, Fonthill Creative

Publishing Manager: Andy Escott

Printed by Mimeo, Huntingdon, Cambridgeshire

Contents

List of contributors

Editors

Tracey A Mills

Lecturer in Midwifery, School of Nursing, Midwifery and Social Work, University of Manchester. Tracey has an interest in care of women with complications of pregnancy. Her PhD focused on investigating placental vascular dysfunction in pregnancies complicated by pre-eclampsia and fetal growth restriction. Her current research focuses on improving care for women of advanced maternal age and parents who have experienced perinatal death.

Debbie M Smith

Health Psychology Lecturer, School of Psychological Sciences, University of Manchester. Debbie's PhD focused on the role of deprivation on young parents' antenatal and postnatal decisions. She has worked in midwifery research for the last four years and has an interest in the antenatal and postnatal period, in particular the opportunity for behaviour change and the role of socio-economic factors.

Dame Tina Lavender

Professor of Midwifery, University of Manchester and Central Manchester Foundation Trust. Dame Tina leads a programme of research around midwifery and women's health. She is Editor of the *British Journal of Midwifery*, Associate Editor of the *Africa Journal of Midwifery and Women's Health*, and on the Editorial team of the *British Journal of Obstetrics and Gynaecology* and Pregnancy and Childbirth group of the Cochrane Collaboration.

Contributors

Carol Bedwell

Lecturer in Midwifery, University of Manchester. Since qualifying as a midwife in 1991 Carol has gained considerable clinical experience, particularly in the area of intrapartum care. She has a wide range of research interests and experience, both in quantitative and qualitative research.

Debra Bick

Professor of Evidence-Based Midwifery Practice, King's College London. Prior to this post, Debra worked at the University of Birmingham, where she completed her master's and doctoral studies, and the Royal College of Nursing. Her research interests include maternal physical and psychological morbidity and approaches to evidence synthesis and translation.

Katherine E Brown

Reader in E-Health and Wellbeing Interventions jointly at Coventry University and Public Health Warwickshire. Katherine is a health psychologist with expertise in the development and evaluation of interventions designed to improve health and wellbeing. She leads the Studies in Adolescent Sexual Health (SASH) research team within the Applied Research Centre at Coventry, which specialises in use of electronic media to deliver sexual health interventions.

Christian Cerra

Academic Foundation Trainee, University Hospital of South Manchester. Christian was educated in Rome, Italy and graduated in pathology (BSc) and medicine (MBChB) from the University of Manchester, UK. His research interest is fertility and reproductive medicine.

Alison Cooke

Part-time Research Midwife in the Maternal and Fetal Health Research Centre, St Mary's Hospital, Manchester/University of Manchester, and part-time Parent Education Midwife at East Cheshire NHS Trust. Her research interests include advanced maternal age, intrapartum care and baby skincare.

Alexander Heazell

Clinical Lecturer in Obstetrics, Maternal and Fetal Health Research Centre, University of Manchester. After graduation from the University of Birmingham Medical School in 2000, Alexander commenced clinical training in obstetrics and gynaecology. After completing his PhD thesis on placenta dysfunction in pre-eclampsia, he has focused his research interests around stillbirth and fetal growth restriction. He is particularly interested in the role that placental dysfunction plays in these conditions. His research portfolio includes a profile of basic science, clinical and qualitative research studies related to understanding and preventing stillbirths and improving care for parents whose babies die before birth.

Lucy Higgins

Clinical Research Fellow, Maternal and Fetal Health Research Centre, University of Manchester. Lucy graduated from the University of Birmingham in 2006 and undertook an academic clinical fellowship in obstetrics and gynaecology in the North West Postgraduate Medical Deanery in 2008 working on placental function in maternal obesity. She is currently undertaking a PhD attempting to identify predictors of poor pregnancy outcome in pregnancies complicated by reduced fetal movements.

Rebecca Lee Jones
Lecturer in Maternal and Fetal Health, University of Manchester. Rebecca's research is on the causes of poor pregnancy outcome in teenage pregnancies, focusing on interactions between maternal age and nutritional status.

Carol Mackay
Senior Lecturer in Midwifery, Coventry University. Carol has a special interest in women's sexual health with experience of working clinically and leading educational programmes in contraception and sexual health care.

Fiona L Mackie
Foundation doctor. Fiona graduated from the University of Manchester Medical School in 2011. In 2010 she completed an Intercalated Masters in Research (with distinction) in Maternal and Fetal Health which she undertook at St Mary's Maternal and Fetal Research Centre.

Julie Elizabeth Maddocks
Assistant Director, Greater Manchester Children's, Young People and Families' NHS Network. Julie qualified as a nurse in 1986 and midwife in 1988. In 2002, she became the Cheshire and Mersey Regional Manager for the Confidential Enquiry into Stillbirth and Death in Infancy (CESDI). In 2003, she became the North West Regional Manager for the Confidential Enquiry into Maternal and Child Health (CEMACH). In 2009 her responsibility extended to the West Midlands and Wales after the establishment of the Centre for Maternal and Child Health (CMACE), which superseded CEMACH.

Lamiya Mohiyiddeen
Sub-specialty Trainee in Reproductive Medicine, St Mary's Hospital, Manchester. Lamiya graduated with MBBS from Manipal Academy of Higher Education in India. She completed Specialist Registrar training in Obstetrics and Gynaecology from the Northwestern Deanery and is a member of the Royal College of Obstetricians and Gynaecologists. Her research interest is in reproductive medicine and she was awarded an MD by the University of Manchester.

Aleksandra Staneva
Research Assistant, University of Manchester. Aleksandra's areas of interest are in perinatal psychology, maternal mental health and mother-infant research.

Sue Thompson
Registered General Nurse. Sue did her nurse training in 1984 and qualified as a midwife in 1986. She has vast experience of providing maternity care to young parents and has worked with young people since 2001. This work includes supporting young dads-to-be. Sue works at Liverpool Victoria Women's Hospital.

Melissa K Whitworth

Consultant Obstetrician, St Mary's Hospital, Central Manchester and Manchester Children's University Hospitals NHS Foundation Trust. Melissa's main areas of interest are substance misuse in pregnancy, teenage pregnancy and the impacts of social deprivation on pregnancy. She was a member of the Guideline Development Group for the NICE Guideline on Socially Complex Pregnancy.

Anja Wittkowski

Lecturer in Clinical Psychology, Clinical Psychology Training Programme, University of Manchester. Anja works part-time as a chartered clinical psychologist for the Mother and Baby Psychiatric Inpatient Unit at Wythenshawe Hospital, Manchester Mental Health and Social Care Trust. She specialises in perinatal clinical psychology.

Lorna Wood

Lead Midwife for Public Health/Vulnerable Women, Liverpool Women's Hospital. Lorna qualified as a registered general nurse in 1983, as a midwife in 1986, and completed a BA Hons in Health Studies in 1992 and a PhD in 2010. She has a particular interest in high risk pregnancy/vulnerable women and developed the first specialist antenatal services for pregnant teenagers in Liverpool.

Foreword

The landscape of pregnancy and motherhood has changed greatly over the past decade. As a result, mortality rates have doubled in the past six years; there were just under 20 deaths per 1000 births in 2010–2011 compared to just under 10 in 2005. Health professionals are being asked to provide maternity care for women with increasingly complex problems, including older first time mothers and teenagers.

The aim of this book is to explore the issues and challenges facing maternity care providers as a result of the changing maternal age profile in the UK. A multidisciplinary team of leading practitioners presents detailed analyses and practical advice to guide midwives, doctors and other professionals when caring for women at extremes of maternal age. A holistic approach is taken and the full range of relevant issues from fertility and contraception to long-term psychosocial needs is covered. Each chapter covers an important aspect of maternity care and provides up-to-date evidence underpinning clinical practice and a discussion of the clinical challenges inherent in providing sensitive and effective antenatal and postnatal care. In a unique approach, each chapter examines issues from the perspectives of both younger and older pregnant women. Clinical scenarios and discussion questions are included to reinforce important concepts and guide learning.

This book provides excellent guidance on the problems older first time mothers and younger mothers are likely to experience. As health professionals it is only when we have this information that we are able to prepare and educate the women in our care.

Yana Richens OBE
Supervisor of Midwives, NICE Fellow, Consultant Midwife University College London Hospitals NHS Trust

Chapter 1

Introduction

Debbie M Smith and Tracey A Mills

Introduction

The rate of teenage pregnancies in the UK remains high, despite a slow decline in recent years (Department for Education, 2012) and pregnancy in women of advanced maternal age is becoming increasingly common, with births to women over 40 increasing three-fold since 1989 (Office for National Statistics, 2010). This trend towards extremes of maternal age is of considerable clinical and public health concern, because both teenage pregnancy and pregnancy at advanced maternal age are associated with increased risks of poor pregnancy outcomes and increased complications during pregnancy and birth. Therefore, reducing the risk of adverse outcomes for younger and older women and their babies remains a significant challenge to maternity services and health professionals.

Teenage pregnancy

The under-18 conception rates in England decreased by 24% between 1998 and 2010; 46.6 per 1000 girls conceived in 1998 compared to 35.4 per 1000 girls in 2010 (Department for Education, 2012). In addition, the number of under-18 conceptions resulting in a live birth decreased by 35%; from 26.9 per 1000 in 1998 to 17.6 per 1000 girls aged 15–17 in 2010 (Department for Education, 2012). Regional and local variations were evident, the North East of England had the highest under-18 conception rate (44.3 per 1000 girls aged 15–17) and the South East had the lowest rate (28.3 per 1000 girls aged 15–17; Department for Education, 2012). Therefore, care must be taken to ensure that the national decrease does not mask any local differences, especially increases in under-18 conception rates, since evidence suggests that the number of young parents presenting for maternity care in England remains high in certain regions of the country. The issues associated with being pregnant aged under 18 and the needs of young parents must be understood and addressed by health professionals at all stages of maternity care if the best maternal and fetal outcomes are to be achieved.

There is an extensive literature examining the psychosocial, cultural and environmental factors associated with poor sexual health and risky health behaviours (see Ingham and Smith, 2009). There is considerable overlap between the reported risk factors for and adverse outcomes of young pregnancy (e.g. low level of qualifications and poor school attendance; Department for Education and Skills, 2007). This complex relationship is unclear. The adverse outcomes associated with young pregnancy are not solely a result of age, but rather an amalgamation of issues, including pre-existing risk factors. Research conducted with this view aims to understand the '…cycle of deprivation…' evident in young pregnancy (Garlick et al, 1993: 139). The influence of social inequalities on outcomes should be central to health services research, particularly given the widening gap between rich and poor (e.g. Dorling et al, 2007). Social inequality exists in young pregnancy, with higher conception prevalence rates and a lower proportion of abortion in more deprived areas relative to more affluent areas (Uren et al, 2007). Research must address the means through which the deprivation of an area relates to individual outcomes as it is difficult to separate the effects of environment from individual circumstances (McCulloch, 2001). Echoing this complexity, Smith and Elander (2006) explored the contributions of geographical area and personal risk factors for sexual behaviour and young pregnancy, concluding that the impact of living in a more deprived area is dependent on individual characteristics. The association between young pregnancy and socioeconomic environment is poorly understood, and mechanisms and processes through which the socioeconomic environment shapes and influences young people's individual sexual and reproductive behaviours are unclear (e.g. Arai, 2007, Smith and Roberts, 2009a, b). The influence of place on sexual and reproductive health needs further exploration (Smith and Roberts, 2011).

The Teenage Pregnancy Strategy was devised as a result of the Social Exclusion Unit report on teenage pregnancy (Social Exclusion Unit, 1999). The report presented young pregnancy as a public health issue by highlighting the greater risk of adverse outcomes for young parents and their children (e.g. social exclusion) and the cost to public spending. In summary, the strategy had two main targets, to reduce the under-18 conception rate by 50% by 2010 and to reduce teenage parents' risk of long-term social exclusion by getting 60% back into education, training or employment. In 2010, the Government produced a report, *Teenage pregnancy strategy: Beyond 2010* (Department for Children, Schools and Families, 2010). This report outlined the successes of the strategy and the plans to take it forward, and these will be discussed in *Chapter 2,* Section 1.

Health professionals are an important feature of the multidisciplinary approach needed to help young parents make informed decisions during the antenatal and postnatal periods. Health professionals must be aware of the increased antenatal risks and complications that are associated with pregnancy at a young age (*Chapter 3*, Section 1). The experience of working with young parents can be a long and time-consuming process. Trust has to be gained, meaning numerous visits, which take time and may not be possible in the current healthcare pathways. To build trust in a shorter period of time will mean listening to the young parents' concerns and needs without judgement, and being knowledgeable about the services that are available to them and to which they can be referred for additional support. If adverse outcomes for young parents and their children are going to decrease, health professionals must engage with young parents and offer them care that meets their antenatal (*Chapter 4*, Section 1) and postnatal needs (*Chapter 5*). Health professionals must also be aware of the possible long-term impact of a pregnancy at an early age for both mother and baby (*Chapter 6*, Section 1).

Advanced maternal age

Delaying or continuing childbearing past the age of 35 is becoming increasingly common among UK women. Recent data from the Office for National Statistics demonstrated that the mean age for giving birth had increased from 28.4 years in 1999 to 29.4 years in 2009. While overall fertility declined slightly over the same period, fertility rates among women aged 35 to 39 years and 40 plus increased by 1% and 2.4%, respectively. Births to women over 40 have nearly trebled in the last 30 years, from 9336 in 1989 to 26976 in 2009 (Office for National Statistics, 2010; *Figure 1.1*). This accelerating demographic shift appears to be a worldwide phenomenon, at least in developed countries. Between 1970 and 2006, the proportion of first births to women over 35 in the USA increased eight-fold (Luke and Brown, 2007). Births to women over 35 accounted for 25% of the total in Australia in 2006 (Australian Bureau of Statistics, 2007).

The trend towards postponement of motherhood has attracted significant concern among health professionals (and others) because of the negative impacts of advancing maternal age on fertility and pregnancy outcomes. Epidemiological studies consistently report increased infertility, miscarriage and need for assisted reproductive technologies in women over 35 (Nybo Andersen et al, 2000), with the real possibility of involuntary childlessness for women who delay motherhood. Older women who sustain a pregnancy are also more likely to experience complications and adverse maternal and perinatal outcomes, notably stillbirth (Cleary-Goldman et al, 2005; Reddy et al 2006; Luke and Brown, 2007). In response to increasing concerns of their members and other health professionals,

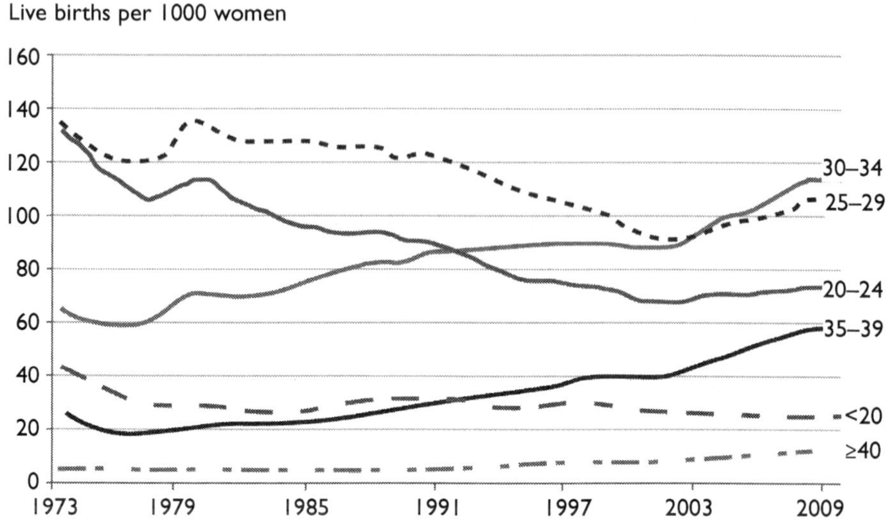

Figure 1.1: Age-specific fertility rates 1973–2009. Source: Office for National Statistics, licensed under the Open Government Licence v 1.0.

the Royal College of Obstetricians and Gynaecologists recently issued a statement encouraging women to '...consider having families during the period of optimal fertility (age 20–35)' (Royal College of Obstetricians and Gynaecologists, 2009).

Provision of effective maternity care to the meet the needs of the increasing number of women becoming pregnant later in life relies on a clear understanding of the risks. However, interpretation of the available evidence is complicated by conflicting data and lack of consensus regarding the magnitude and importance of particular risks. Investigation of the effect of age on (fortunately) infrequent outcomes such as stillbirth requires a large sample. Although births to older women are becoming more common, they account for a small percentage of the total, around 10–20% births are to women over 35 and 2–4% to women over 40. The largest studies are based on retrospective examinations of birth registers which may lack data on many variables that could significantly influence outcome. For example, the children of older women may be fathered by older men. Older women also have an increased incidence of co-existing medical conditions, are more likely to be primiparous, use assisted reproductive technologies including ovarian stimulation/*in vitro* fertilisation and have multiple pregnancies. All of these are independent risk factors for poor pregnancy outcome. The age range of the control groups used for comparison also varies considerably between studies (examples include 20–30, 25–29, and under 35 years) (Nybo Andersen et al, 2000; Reddy et al, 2006).

The limitations present in many of the existing studies reduce the validity and generalisability of findings (Kenyon and Bewley, 2009), meaning that many key questions remain unanswered. It is not clear whether increased risks of poor outcome relate to maternal age *per se* or the presence of co-morbidities. Evidence relating to the age threshold at which adverse outcomes become significant is also limited. Some studies have suggested this occurs after 35 years, while others argue that the association is only clinically important at age 40.

Despite the evidence for worsening reproductive outcomes, the trend towards delaying childbearing shows no signs of slowing. The reasons underlying this phenomenon are incompletely understood but shifting gender roles, increased independence and an emphasis on the importance of education and career for women are often cited. Access to effective contraception, assisted reproductive technologies and changing patterns of family building, including increased divorce rates and remarriage, are also likely to contribute (Carolan and Frankowska, 2011). Surprisingly, there has been little empirical research to examine women's reasoning and views concerning the timing of childbearing. A recent qualitative study challenges the assumption that women perceive delayed childbearing as a conscious choice (Cooke et al, 2012). In Cooke and colleagues' study, women who had delayed motherhood past the age of 35, identified a complex interplay of personal, social, economic and cultural factors as constraining earlier childbearing.

Despite the negative focus on an apparent increase in physical risks, later childbearing may have some advantages for the mother and baby. Childbearing women aged over 35 are likely to be better educated and of higher socioeconomic status than in the past. Older women may be more likely to follow a healthy lifestyle, attend for regular antenatal care and have a positive perception of their pregnancy, factors that are strongly associated with lower rates of poor outcome. Women in their 30s and 40s will also have greater life experience and information, which may mean that they feel more psychologically prepared to assume the responsibilities of parenthood. A recent Canadian study also identified a strong association of older maternal age and prolonged breastfeeding (Kehler et al, 2009). However, there is some evidence that older women might experience greater difficulties in adjusting to the demands of caring for a newborn infant in the early postnatal period. Bornstein et al (2006) reported that increasing maternal age is correlated to perception of the newborn as 'difficult' or maladjusted, possibly reflecting a decline in physical capacity and stamina with advancing age. Older women may also lack social support from extended families, which often benefits younger women. While there are relatively few data regarding outcomes for the children of older mothers, there appears to be no evidence of any negative effect of maternal age on children's psychosocial wellbeing. One study reported that advanced maternal age was the strongest predictor of high educational achievement and positive psychosocial development in young adults at the age of 18 years (Fergusson and Woodward, 1999).

Summary

Providing effective, sensitive care requires an understanding of the unique issues and challenges affecting pregnant women at both ends of the age spectrum. Health professionals and maternity service providers need to understand the impact of maternal age on the health and wellbeing of pregnant women, their babies and their own parents. They must also be aware of recent policy recommendations for care and the most effective strategies to reduce the impact of associated complications.

References

Australian Bureau of Statistics (2007) *Births Australia, 2006*. Australian Government Press, Canberra

Arai L (2007) Peer and neighbour influences on teenage pregnancy and fertility: Qualitative findings from research in English communities. *Health and Place* **13**: 87–98

Bornstein MH, Putnick DL, Suwalsky, JT, Gini M (2006) Maternal chronological age, prenatal and perinatal history, social support, and parenting of infants. *Child Development* **77**(4): 875–92

Carolan M, Frankowska D (2011) Advanced maternal age and adverse perinatal outcome: A review of the evidence. *Midwifery* **27**(6): 793–801

Cleary-Goldman JFD, Malone J, Vidaver RH, et al (2005) Impact of maternal age on obstetric outcome. *Obstetrics and Gynecology* **105**(5 Pt 1): 983–90

Cooke A, Mills TA, Lavender, T (2012) Advanced maternal age: Delayed childbearing is rarely a conscious choice. A qualitative study of women's views and experiences. *International Journal of Nursing Studies* **49**(1): 30–9

Department for Children, Schools and Families (2010) *Teenage pregnancy strategy: Beyond 2010*. Department for Children, Schools and Families, Nottingham

Department for Education (2012) *Under-18 conception statistics; 1998–2010*. Available from: http://media.education.gov.uk/assets/files/pdf/u/under-18%20and%20under-16%20conceptions%202010%20-%20key%20findings.pdf

Department for Education and Skills (2007) *Improving access to sexual health services for young people in further education settings*. The Stationery Office, London

Dorling D, Rigby J, Wheeler B, et al (2007) *Poverty, wealth and place in Britain, 1968 to 2005*. The Policy Press, Bristol, UK

Fergusson DM, Woodward LJ (1999) Maternal age and educational and psychosocial outcomes in early adulthood. *Journal of Child Psychology and Psychiatry* **40**: 479–89

Garlick R, Ineichen B, Hudson F (1993) The UPA score and teenage pregnancy. *Public Health* **107**: 135–9

Ingham R, Smith D (2009) Vulnerability and sexual health. In Killoran A, Kelly M (eds) *Effectiveness and efficiency in public health: Systematic approaches to evidence and practice* (pp 79–96). NICE/OUP collaboration, London

Kehler HL, Chaput KH, Tough SC (2009) Risk factors for cessation of breastfeeding prior to six months postpartum among a community sample of women in Calgary, Alberta. *Canandian Journal of Public Health* **100**(5): 376–80

Kenyon A, Bewley S (2009) The effect of age on obstetric (maternal and fetal) outcomes. In Bewley S, Ledger WL, Nikolaou D (eds) *Reproductive aging* (pp 125–40). RCOG Press, London

Luke B, Brown MB (2007) Contemporary risks of maternal morbidity and adverse outcomes with increasing maternal age and plurality. *Fertility and Sterility* **88**(2): 283–93

McCulloch A (2001) Teenage childbearing in Great Britain and the spatial concentration of poverty households. *Journal of Epidemiology and Community Health* **55**: 16–23

Nybo Andersen AM, Wohlfahrt J, Christens P et al (2000) Maternal age and fetal loss: Population-based register linkage study. *British Medical Journal* **320**(7251): 1708–12

Office for National Statistics (2010) *Statistical Bulletin: Births and Deaths in England and Wales 2009*. Office for National Statistics, Newport

Royal College of Obstetricians and Gynaecologists (2009) *Statement on later maternal age*. Available from: http://www.rcog.org.uk/what-we-do/campaigning-and-opinions/statement/rcog-statement-later-maternal-age [Accessed 16 May 2011]

Reddy UM, Ko CW, Willinger M (2006) Maternal age and the risk of stillbirth throughout pregnancy in the United States. *American Journal of Obstetrics and Gynecology* **195**(3): 764–70

Smith DM, Elander J (2006) Effects of area and family deprivation on risk factors for teenage pregnancy among 13–15-year-old girls. *Psychology, Health and Medicine* **11**(4): 399–410

Smith DM, Roberts R (2009a) Young parents' perceptions of barriers to antenatal and postnatal care. *British Journal of Midwifery* **17**(10): 620–7

Smith DM, Roberts R (2009b) Social acceptance; a possible mediator in the association between socio-economic deprivation and under-18 pregnancy rates? *Journal of Youth Studies* **12**(6): 669–83

Smith DM, Roberts R (2011) Social inequality and young pregnancy; the causal attributions of young parents in London, UK. *Health and Place* **17**: 1054–60

Social Exclusion Unit (1999) *Teenage pregnancy*. Her Majesty's Stationary Office, London

Uren Z, Sheers D, Dattani N (2007) Teenage conceptions by small area deprivation in England and Wales, 2001–2002. *Health Statistics Quarterly* **33**: 34–9

Chapter 2

Preconception issues and public health

Introduction

This chapter outlines specific preconception issues relevant to the care of teenagers and women of advanced maternal age. A public health approach is taken with a discussion of implications for clinical practice and public policy. *Section 1* considers the Teenage Pregnancy Strategy, with a focus on its impact in reducing teenage pregnancy and associated poor outcomes, and the future of public policy in this area. *Section 2* addresses the effects of aging on fertility and issues surrounding provision, practice and ethics of fertility treatment for women of advanced maternal age.

Section 1
Vulnerable young people and the Teenage Pregnancy Strategy: Beyond 2010

Katherine E Brown and Carol MacKay

Introduction

Some young people, particularly those from lower socioeconomic groups and deprived backgrounds, are at high risk of under-18 conception (planned and unplanned), as well as other outcomes that are relevant to their broader health and wellbeing. The Teenage Pregnancy Strategy (TPS; Social Exclusion Unit, 1999) set out to address prevention and support on this issue, and ultimately to reduce the rate of under-18 conception by half, by 2010. The *Teenage Pregnancy Strategy: Beyond 2010* report (Department of Health and Department for Children, Schools and Families, 2010) was published shortly before the then Labour Government lost power to a Conservative–Liberal Democrat coalition in May 2010. At the time of writing, the Coalition Government has not produced plans specifically to address teenage pregnancy, and seems unlikely to do so, since the publication of *Improving behaviour, changing outcomes: A new social marketing strategy for public health* (Department of Health, 2011) where they advocate a life course marketing approach to health rather than a topic-driven approach. Traditionally,

Department of Health public health campaigns have focused on a single issue (e.g. alcohol misuse). It is recognised that this approach fails to acknowledge the links between health risk behaviours. A life course marketing approach aims to deliver support on all health topics relevant to people at particular life stages. A Department of Health sexual health policy document is due for publication, in the near future.

In light of this, this chapter explains some of the factors associated with under-18 conception, and draws on recent relevant policy documents and some of the preventive strategies set out in *TPS: Beyond 2010* to summarise current and recent political thinking targeted at preventing under-18 conception in the UK. Some critique of the original Labour-led plans is provided, highlighting what was good, but also what was lacking. The way the current Government appears to be adopting and developing some of these ideas is explained. The coalition Government's interest in insights from behavioural science in leading policy making, the impact of the Marmot Review (Marmot et al, 2010) and findings from the broader evidence base, are drawn on to make the case for the way forward. It is argued this must include a greater translation of behaviour change approaches and a focus on addressing social inequalities and broader health and wellbeing issues in preconception prevention work with young people. A case study and some examples of applications of an evidence-based approach to implementing TPS recommendations are provided to help illustrate the arguments made.

Vulnerable young people

Teenagers by definition are a vulnerable group. During adolescence, young people make the transition from childhood to adulthood, coping with, among other things, their changing bodies and awakening sexuality. Within Western cultures, developing adolescents may challenge authority and parental control to some extent, and place greater value on the opinions of their peer group (Reyna and Farley, 2006). Risk-taking is a feature of this phase of development and it is argued that from an evolutionary perspective the tendency to take risks is necessary to enable the young to leave their childhood home (Reyna and Farley, 2006). Emotional cognitive processing develops faster than rational processing at this time, and dominates cognition (Steinberg, 2008). This tends to mean that experimentation and thrill-seeking are more common in this age group than among adults, and adolescents are more likely to engage in risky experiences that provide immediate reward than evaluate risk and act according to more rational judgements (Department of Health, 2011).

Risk-taking behaviours, including sexual risk-taking, have an impact on the health of young people. In recent decades there have been overall improvements in health outcomes in all age groups except adolescence (Viner and Barker, 2005). Smoking, drug use and alcohol are all documented as having adverse effects on health and obstetric outcomes (Chen et al, 2007). Although cigarette smoking and drug use has decreased among 11–19 year olds over the last 25 years (Coleman and Brooks, 2009) as has the proportion of young people who drink, the levels of alcohol consumed have increased significantly over the last decade (Fuller, 2011). Both smoking and drinking at a young age increase the likelihood of engaging in unprotected sex (Jayakodi et al, 2005).

Although adolescents in general can be considered more likely to engage in risk-taking behaviour and more vulnerable to certain adverse health outcomes, there are particular subgroups of this population at greatest risk. Young people from lower socioeconomic groups and deprived backgrounds are more likely than their more advantaged counterparts to engage in risk-taking behaviour, such as smoking and drinking, to have started having sex by age 16 years, to engage in risky sexual behaviour, and to become pregnant aged under 19 years (Social Exclusion Unit, 1999; Jayakodi et al, 2005; Department for Education and Skills, 2006; Department of Health and Department for Children, Schools & Families, 2010). Low self-esteem in young women increases the risk of engaging in unprotected sex (Jayakodi et al, 2005) and young people from lower socioeconomic groups are also more likely to express wanting to become parents at a young age (Newby, 2011b).

In addition to these broader risk factors, research has found teenagers living in seaside areas are affected by a carnivalised atmosphere that appears to be associated with a suspension of everyday life and a greater likelihood of engaging in casual sex (Bell et al, 2004), and those in rural areas have identified sexual health services as being 'too visible' and inaccessible (Bell et al, 2004). Young people in care, those who are homeless, involved in crime or from some minority ethnic groups also appear to be particularly vulnerable (Health Development Agency, 2003). Adolescents' abilities to avoid or manage risk are strongly associated with having good social support networks, higher socioeconomic status and family and school connectedness (Jayakodi et al, 2005; Brooks et al, 2011). Parent–child closeness and a stable or intact family structure and/or having a positive relationship with an adult family member to access for advice, are also protective (Scott et al, 2011).

Clearly, the relationship between factors associated with adverse health outcomes and risky behaviour among young people is complex, and therefore difficult to address. This will be discussed later in relation to the TPS. In addition, although it is somewhat beyond the scope of this chapter, it is worth noting that risky sexual behaviour and adverse health and wellbeing outcomes associated with conception are strongly related to wider health issues of young people. Those involved with young people in sexual health and prevention work are well placed to consider how the substantive arguments and approaches outlined below might also help address broader health and wellbeing issues.

TPS: Beyond 2010

The *TPS: Beyond 2010* report outlines progress made to date in reducing teenage pregnancy since the strategy began. It concedes that the 13% reduction demonstrable in the 2008 data (Office for National Statistics, 2010a) does not make it likely that the intended target of a 50% reduction by 2010 will be achieved (the 2010 data released in 2012 have shown a 15% reduction in England since TPS began; Office for National Statistics, 2012). In addition, the 13% reduction is a national average and while there are areas in the country that have shown quite significant rates of reduction (28% of areas report more than a 20% reduction), around 14% of areas report an increase since the strategy began (Department of Health and Department for Children, Schools and Families, 2010). Furthermore, although the TPS report does not mention it, there is evidence that rates of under-18 conception were falling anyway at a similar rate in the years before the strategy was introduced (Wellings and Kane, 1999). There is therefore a clear need to reflect on the efficacy of the strategy beyond 2010.

The social and economic benefits of tackling teenage pregnancy are also explicated, drawing on the link between this issue and socioeconomic deprivation. The case is made that there are two factors that have the strongest impact on reducing teenage pregnancy rates (based on a review not yet published at the time of the report). First is good quality curriculum-based sex and relationships education (SRE). SRE is the term used in the TPS report but more recently there has been a shift to use relationships and sex education (RSE), placing greater importance on relationships rather than sex in the phrase. Second is the provision of '…accessible, young person-centred contraception and sexual health (CASH) services' (Department of Health and Department of Children, Schools and Families, 2010: 17). Whilst providing good RSE and quality CASH services for young people is undoubtedly important, there are two points at issue here. First, the case for the causal relationship between teenage pregnancy and health inequalities and child poverty is somewhat overstated. These issues are strongly associated with one another, but becoming pregnant under 18 is not the direct or sole cause of poorer health outcomes and poverty (Luker, 2000; Baker et al, 2007). Rather, these issues are intertwined in a complex interplay of causality and interdependence. Arguably, rates of under-18 conception and childbirth can be seen as a metric of inequality and social deprivation and a clear case can be made for needing to tackle these issues simultaneously. Second, although there is good evidence of the importance of well-designed and delivered RSE and CASH services, in focusing on these two factors, the strategy fails to address fully the complexity of the issue. The evidence that knowledge is necessary but not sufficient for supporting people consistently to behave in ways that are beneficial to their health and wellbeing has been well established (e.g. Abraham et al, 2002; Conner and Norman, 2005; Allen et al, 2007; Brown et al, 2011). Complex social, environmental and cultural factors interact with individual psychosocial factors in determining decision-making and action relevant to sexual and contraceptive behaviours. Thus, although a young person may have sufficient knowledge about contraception and where and how to get hold of it and use it properly, there may be a range of other determinants of his/her behaviour that supersede this. *Case study 2.1* illustrates some of the relevant wider influences on an instance of under-16 conception in the West Midlands.

Case study 2.1

Nicky is a 17-year-old young woman who became pregnant aged 15. The baby was unplanned but she proceeded with the pregnancy and has a girl aged 8 months. She is still in a relationship with the father (Andy) who is 18 years old and unemployed; he was 16 when Nicky conceived. Nicky lives at home with her mother (Sue), three of her six siblings, and the baby. Her parents are separated and her mother, who is aged between 40 and 49, describes herself as a 'lapsed Catholic'. Nicky is studying for A-levels and hopes to go on to further education to study languages.

Despite being academic and achieving at school, Nicky was disengaged with education prior to conception. She reports finding school boring and having lots of days off. Nicky describes herself as uncomfortable talking about sex and both her mother and Andy acknowledge this. Her mother's approach to sex education has been to provide open and honest answers to questions from her children and has even gone as far as providing a condom demonstration. She has also used opportunities to put across important messages. However, Nicky does not recall at any time having, what she calls, a 'proper conversation'. Nicky remembers having some sex education at school but can't remember any specifics. She doesn't recall learning anything in particular and commented that she would have liked more information on relationships, but is unable to elaborate on what.

At the age of 13 (when Nicky first had sex in an earlier relationship), and up to the point of conception, she was mixing with a promiscuous peer group. She also had a further peer group who were not so interested in boys and were more academic. She met Andy whilst socialising/drinking at the Cathedral where she sometimes stayed until late at night. Nicky's mum (Sue) didn't like this behaviour but did not monitor it, enjoying her daughter's popularity (a consequence of an older daughter having been bullied). She now regrets allowing her daughter so much freedom, as does Nicky who believes that if her mum had imposed greater restrictions she would not have got pregnant (because of having less time to spend with Andy). Within a few weeks of meeting, Nicky and Andy had had sex (unprotected) for the first time (influenced by alcohol). Andy had had several previous sexual partners. Neither partner reports feeling pressured into having sex and Nicky remembers them agreeing that they should use condoms. Neither Nicky nor Andy was at all confident purchasing condoms; Nicky never bought them but Andy accessed them from shops in town (e.g. Sainsbury's) and occasionally from Connexions. Andy didn't like getting them from Connexions because of the wait which prolonged embarrassment. Nicky reports preferring to get them from shops which she felt was more grown-up.

Nicky was initially highly motivated to use condoms and feared getting pregnant. However, as the relationship progressed the occasional non-use of condoms led to decreased feelings of susceptibility and both even suspected that they may be infertile (despite Andy having previously fathered a child). Neither partner took responsibility for ensuring condoms were always available and when they weren't, this did not prevent sex happening. On occasions when they didn't use condoms they used withdrawal.

Sue strongly suspected that Nicky and Andy were having sex (aware of Nicky's previous sexual relationship). She asked her daughter directly but this was denied. Nicky describes her mother's approach as saying, 'You best not be doing it'. Sue also told Nicky's uncles about her suspicions and they teased her saying, 'Don't be a little slag'.

Andy was homeless during this period, having been thrown out by his mother, and was 'sofa hopping' between friends' houses. Nicky describes it as always being easier to meet where Andy was staying (presumably due to lack of monitoring). They had access to a house belonging to the father of a friend who was 'never there' and they often met there with a group of friends and stayed the night.

Questions and discussion points

- What do you think are the key contributing factors to Nicky becoming pregnant?
- How can these factors be categorised? Are they psychological, interpersonal, cultural, environmental or other types?
- Nicky's mother has given Nicky information about condom use and answers her questions. Do you feel this was appropriate? If not, why? Can you suggest how this topic could be handled by Nicky's mother?
- How do you think health and social care professionals could contribute to supporting Nicky to continue in education and avoid a further pregnancy?

Reproduced with permission from Newby K (2009) *Under-16 conceptions in the West Midlands: An investigation. Final Report for Government Office West Midlands*

Clearly, every instance of unintended adolescent conception is unique, but *Case study 2.1* illustrates some of the relevant broader socioeconomic, cultural and environmental influences, including Andy's NEET (not in employment, education or training) status and homelessness, a sexually promiscuous peer group, as well as more direct interpersonal and psychosocial influences. For example, despite Sue's apparent openness for communication about sex and condom use, embarrassment on Nicky's part and a lack of communication about Nicky's actual situation and feelings seem likely to have influenced the outcome here. In addition, Nicky and Andy's beliefs about susceptibility to pregnancy, and embarrassment and difficulties associated with access to condoms, appear to have had a direct impact on their limited use by the couple over time. Arguably, strategy and approaches to address teenage conception need to target all of these kinds of determinants to be effective (see the questions and discussion points for *Case study 2.1*).

The Marmot Review, published shortly before the Government came to power (Marmot et al, 2010), the Coalition's programme for government report (HM Government, 2010a), their recent public health report (HM Government, 2010b), and the House of Lords' Behaviour Change report (House of Lords, 2011) demonstrate some of the broader political thinking relevant to this issue. The Marmot Review, which has been well received and influential on thinking around public health strategy (HM Government, 2010b), explored the issue of health inequalities in England and outlined a set of six policy objectives aimed at addressing inequality, including giving children the best start in life and enabling people of all ages to maximise their capabilities and have control over their lives. Health inequalities and teenage conception are part of the same broad picture of social issues, and arguably, if the objectives set out by Marmot are embedded within policymaking effectively, there ought to be an impact on some of the wider determinants of teenage conception as well. In addition, the Coalition have demonstrated an interest in the ways in which policy-making can make better use of the evidence base from the behavioural sciences to influence people's behaviour and improve health outcomes, among other things. They noted an interest in their programme for government in the use of Thaler and Sunstein's (2008) 'nudge' approach (whereby people are steered towards healthy behaviours by changing their environment in such a way that the healthier choices are easy to access and attractive), and have responded to the recent House of Lords Science and Technology Select Committee report on behaviour change. The report had suggested that while the Government's favoured 'nudge' approach is useful, it needs to ensure it draws on a broad range of approaches for influencing behaviour change, makes better use of the evidence in policy design, and ensures that robust evaluation of strategies and policies is undertaken. Arguably, these conclusions also apply to the issue of preventing teenage conception, and some specifics in relation to Chapters 3, 4 and 5 of *TPS: Beyond 2010* are drawn out below.

TPS: Beyond 2010 also sets out the strategy's aims in relation to achieving improvement in young people's knowledge and skills around relationships and sexual health. Some achievements to date are noted, but in addition, aims relating to improving the quality of SRE are set out, making this a statutory part of the curriculum for key stages 1–4. Improving communication between young people and their parents about relationships and sex is also prioritised. The Coalition Government stopped the bill to make personal, social and health education (PSHE) which includes RSE (relationship and sex education), statutory, when they came to power in 2010. They later published broad reforms to public health but made it clear that within the present non-statutory framework, 'schools will provide age-appropriate teaching on relationships and sexual health' (HM Government, 2010b: 34). In the 2011 update report, however, little mention is given to sexual health and there is no mention of PSHE or RSE (HM Government, 2011). Without firm Government commitment to PSHE and RSE it will likely be delivered in an *ad hoc* fashion by schools and regions, leaving some young people with no provision at all.

Despite abandoning plans to make PSHE statutory, the current Government and those involved in implementing strategy should pick up on other TPS recommendations for improving RSE. The original *TPS: Beyond 2010* report included initiatives to give the 'learner' a stronger voice and to assess young people's perceptions of the RSE they receive to make sure that what is delivered meets their needs. These are positive and important aims, and the desire for this from young people is borne out in recent survey research (UK Youth Parliament, 2007). It is also arguably the case, however, that there is a need to go beyond this to ensure that RSE not only meets young people's perceived needs but also involves learning strategies and activities based on evidence about what will be likely to influence their behaviour. Recent research, for example, with 13 to 16-year-old school pupils in England, demonstrated that knowledge about contraception, and pupils' evaluations of their school sex education were entirely unrelated to their intentions to use condoms, intentions to use the contraceptive pill, and intentions to use emergency contraception if something had gone wrong with their normal method (Bayley et al, 2009, 2010). Other research has also demonstrated the relative lack of importance of high levels of knowledge (e.g. Allen et al, 2007). Statistically significant relationships did exist, however, between pupils' attitudes towards using contraceptive methods, their perceptions about what other people in their lives thought they should do, their confidence in their ability to use contraception, with their intentions to use these methods (Bayley et al, 2009, 2010). Intention is known to be a good predictor of health-relevant behaviour (Abraham et al, 2002; Conner and Norman, 2005) and condom use intention predicted condom use among the sexually active young people in this sample (there were not enough data to assess the relationship between intentions and behaviour for the pill or emergency contraception) (Bayley et al, 2009, 2010). This evidence suggests that RSE should aim to go beyond improving knowledge.

Arguably, in order to influence contraceptive behaviour and condom use, the focus should be on enhancing positive attitudes towards contraceptive use, increasing confidence in ability to use condoms and contraception, building positive perceptions about what important others think about the desired behaviours, and what important others do themselves. These ideas are borne out within behaviour change approaches and *Box 2.1* provides more detail about behaviour change. *Behaviour Change Example 2.1* then provides a typical sex education activity, why it may be problematic in influencing behaviour and how it could take account of evidence such as that outlined above, to be more effective.

Whether influenced by behaviour change evidence or not, wherever possible, programmes and the activities they contain need to be evaluated for their impact on behaviour and health-related outcomes. In the TPS report, for example, mention is made of 'the award-winning L8R project', a sex education programme which 'integrates interactive drama on video and the web', and gives 'access to advice

Box 2.1. What is 'behaviour change'?

The science of behaviour change is cross-disciplinary and incorporates, but is not exhaustively inclusive of, the knowledge base from sociology, medicine and psychology. By researching the broad range of factors that influence the way people think and behave, it is both theoretically possible and increasingly empirically demonstrated that we can draw on the scientific evidence base to design interventions to change human behaviour. Given that much of the mortality and morbidity in Western industrialised nations today is caused by human behaviour, there is an increasing need to apply such knowledge to real-world health problems.

Dependent on the factors that are most influential in affecting a given behaviour, effective interventions could be environmental and in the past have included things like a ban on smoking in public places and the introduction of traffic calming measures such as speed bumps. Interventions can also work at the individual level and include techniques such as providing people with information about the consequences of a behaviour, modelling a desired behaviour, or supporting goal setting (see Abraham and Michie, 2008).

Knowing which factors are the most important in influencing a particular behaviour in a particular context and within a particular population is important for selecting the correct techniques for intervention.

and information and online mentoring' (Department of Health and Department for Children, Schools and Families, 2010: 21). The report recognises the programme for its engaging nature but nothing is said about its impact on important outcomes such as the determinants of health-protective behaviour or the sexual health and wellbeing of those who have engaged with it. Much greater emphasis needs to be placed on delivering programmes and curricula that have demonstrated success, and when outcomes are not achieved, efforts must be made to understand why, so that continued efforts are not wasted.

In relation to providing more support to parents in talking to their children about relationships and sex, it is unlikely to be disputed that parents and other important adults in young people's lives have a critical role to play in helping them to make good decisions relevant to their sexual health and wellbeing. This is often something that parents find challenging or avoid altogether (Newby et al, 2011a). The campaign, *Sex: Worth talking about*, is specifically advocated by the TPS report in respect of this issue and this is something that the Coalition Government has picked up on in their publication, *Changing*

Behaviour Change Example 2.1. Condom demonstration

Providing a demonstration of how to put on a condom is a common sex education activity. It seems like a perfectly sensible and rational approach for ensuring young people know how to use condoms. However, knowing *how* to do something and actually *wanting* to do it are not the same thing. Confidence in ability is known to be important in relation to wanting to perform, and actually performing, a range of health-relevant behaviours, including, for some groups at least, condom use.

Although viewing a condom demonstration may have a positive impact on an individual's confidence in their ability to put a condom on, the demonstration is unlikely to have any substantial impact on confidence to perform other important behaviours required for successful condom use, including confidence to access condoms, to carry them, to negotiate their use with a partner or to remove and dispose of them when sex is complete.

Other considerations include the fact that simply watching a condom demonstration performed by an adult may provide a fairly limited mastery experience and not lead to a significant improvement in confidence to use a condom. In addition, if young people are given the opportunity to try the demonstration themselves, there is the potential for the behaviour of others to impact on feelings of confidence. For example, if errors are made and others make fun of or laugh at an individual, confidence may be reduced instead of enhanced. It seems likely that getting young people to work in very small groups or pairs around this activity may be most appropriate.

behaviour, improving outcomes: A new social marketing strategy for public health (Department of Health, 2011). Although the Coalition expects local councils and GP (now known as Clinical Commissioning Groups) consortia to deliver sexual health services solely at a local level from 2013, they intend to provide existing assets, such as those developed for the programme, *Sex: Worth talking about*, for free to local teams to use and adapt as they see fit. The original campaign was based, in part, on evidence for the role of communication in behaviour change (Department of Health and Department of Children, Schools and Families, 2009), but local level initiatives and activities will also need to draw on the evidence and the needs of the particular population or groups with whom they intend to work if they are to have an impact. *Behaviour Change Example 2.2* explains the development of an intervention in Warwickshire and Coventry designed to help parents communicate more effectively with their children about relationships and sex. It was based on the needs of local parents and relevant theory and evidence for behavioural change.

TPS: Beyond 2010 goes on to focus on young people's access to contraception and sexual health (CASH) services. Among the policy-level initiatives is the promotion of the *You're welcome* quality criteria for health services which identify best practice for delivering young-people-friendly health services, including sexual health services. Services are only awarded the *You're welcome*

Behaviour Change Example 2.2. 'What should we tell the children about relationships and sex?' (© What Shall We Tell the Children?)

For a full description of the development process of this intervention, please see Newby et al (2011a).

This intervention had the overall programme objective of improving the quality and quantity of communication between parents and their children about relationships and sex and was developed using a process known as intervention mapping (Bartholomew et al, 2001, 2006, 2011). The programme development began with thorough needs assessment work. This drew on communication with a specially set up community partnership group, focus groups with parents, literature searches and a review of existing parenting programmes. Predisposing, reinforcing and enabling factors associated with parent–child communication on this issue were identified through needs assessment and matched to known determinants of behaviour from the literature that were amenable to change within a parenting programme. These included attitudinal beliefs (e.g. 'My child's not old enough yet'), deficits of skill and knowledge (e.g. 'I don't know where to start') and a lack of confidence in ability (e.g. 'I don't have the ability to influence my child'). Change objectives that targeted determinants of behaviour and aimed at achieving the performance objectives of the programme were identified. Theoretical methods and practical strategies were then selected in collaboration with the community partnership group for inclusion in the programme and parents were consulted to ensure the acceptability of the strategies in the programme. To illustrate this, the link between a single performance objective and a final practical strategy used in the programme follows:

- *Performance objective*: Parents to recognise the scope and importance of relationships and sex education and their role in providing it.
- An example of an attitudinal determinant associated with this performance objective was: It's not my job to talk to my kids about relationships and sex.

- A change objective associated with addressing this determinant was: Develop awareness of the message parents give their children by *not* communicating about relationships and sex.
- A theoretical method selected to address this change objective was: Provide information about consequences.
- A practical strategy selected to deliver this theoretical method was: A group discussion guided by a facilitator and involving parents thinking about the messages conveyed to them about relationships and sex by their own parents and the consequences of that for them.

This programme runs across Coventry and Warwickshire for parents who want to attend. Some parents lack time to do so or are not keen to join in with group programmes. For this reason, an online shortened version of the programme has been designed as a Serious Game and can be accessed and played by parents at www.besavvy.org.uk. A demo of the game, for those interested but not wanting to play the full version, is available at www.healthinterventions.co.uk.

Questions and discussion points

- How could health and social care professionals engage parents on the issue of successful communication with their children about relationships and sex?
- What particular challenges do professionals face in engaging with hard-to-reach groups on this issue and how could they be overcome?
- What level do the challenges exist at: cultural, environmental, psychological, interpersonal, behavioural or others? How can that help you to design better strategies for addressing the problem?

stamp when they have demonstrated they meet the best practice requirements. This involves a range of things, but includes provision of the services young people want, in accessible locations, open at times young people need them, and run by welcoming, non-judgemental staff. The Government is keen to maintain this approach to ensuring services meet the needs of young people, stating that they, 'Should have easy access to health services they trust, for example accredited *You're welcome* young-people-friendly services' (HM Government, 2010b: 35). In relation to this aspect of enhancing provision, activities and initiatives designed to enhance access to sexual health services also need to draw on the evidence base to inform what is done. Evaluation of such activities to assess their impact is also imperative. *Behaviour Change Example 2.3* briefly describes the development and evaluation of an evidence-based smart phone app, aimed at enhancing access to sexual health services under development at the time of writing at NHS Warwickshire.

Behaviour Change Example 2.3.
Smartphone app for enhancing sexual health service access

NHS Warwickshire were keen to develop a smartphone app to support access to sexual health services across Coventry and Warwickshire. They had noted the existence of a local smartphone app that used global positioning software (GPS) to locate users and tell them where their nearest sexual health service was. However, they were concerned that the database it was linked to could not be updated and so sought to develop an app with greater flexibility for the changing nature of services.

Such an app, however, has the potential to do more than simply provide users with information, and the NHS collaborated with researchers to develop one that used behavioural change approaches aimed at enhancing the likelihood that those who use it would act on the information provided. The app, which at the time of writing is under technical development, has been designed using the intervention mapping approach referred to in *Example 2.2*. Needs analysis and literature searching has helped identify the factors that predispose, reinforce and enable young people's access to sexual health services when they have a sexual health issue or need.

The app will be available via ordinary computers with internet access as well as mobile devices and will directly address determinants of behaviour associated with service access. For example, a factor that enables service access is knowing exactly how to get to the service. The app, therefore, will offer information not only about where the service is but also will deliver specifics about exactly how to get there and approximately how much doing so will cost (e.g. in bus fares). Another enabling factor involves young people feeling that their visit is confidential and that no-one they know will see them accessing the service. The app will therefore include a feature to allow them to find the next nearest service if the nearest one is too close to home to allow their visit to remain confidential.

The app is currently being showcased on the Department of Health Maps and Apps web pages (see http://mapsandapps.dh.gov.uk/2011/11/30/coventry-sexual-health/) and is available via www.respectyourself.info. Evaluation of the app will be carried out to assess its impact on service uptake and the factors associated with uptake that it is designed to address. Findings and associated publications will be reported on via www.healthinterventions.co.uk.

Intervening early with those young people who are most at risk of teenage pregnancy is the subject of Chapter 5 in *TPS: Beyond 2010*. Given the link between social and economic deprivation and teenage pregnancy outlined earlier, coupled with conclusions from the Marmot Review about the need to address health inequalities, it is argued that this has to be a major part of the work to reduce under-18 conceptions and address other important health and wellbeing issues in the future.

Using the theory and evidence from behavioural change research is important when the aim is to help individuals feel motivated and develop the skills to use condoms, or enhance the likelihood that young people will take up offers of service provision. However, addressing wider determinants at an early stage may have a greater overall impact. A recent systematic review has shown there is sound evidence that providing social skills and youth development programmes which combine community service and student learning, or a programme of academic and social development is effective at reducing teenage pregnancy (Harden et al, 2006). Statistical meta-analysis demonstrated that these approaches led to a 39% reduction in the number of young women reporting teenage pregnancy, and had a positive impact on employment and economic status (Harden et al, 2006). A further review demonstrated that multifaceted intervention programmes which might include outreach work, engagement of young people in volunteering or use of virtual-world simulations as well as classroom-based education are effective at reducing unintended pregnancies (Oringanje et al, 2009). Targeting these kinds of interventions at young people at risk of teenage pregnancy and/or risky behaviours seems likely to be effective, but basing the specifics of programmes on evidence and ensuring evaluation is robust will remain important. In addition, seeking to have impact years before young people become adolescents, as recommended by Graham Allen MP in his report to the Government entitled *Early intervention: The next steps* (Allen, 2011), seems likely to be beneficial for a wide range of social, emotional, health and wellbeing issues for the most vulnerable in society. In accordance with a key line of argument in this chapter, Allen (2011) also stresses the importance of robust evaluation of early intervention work, and the need to engage in review and expansion of what is delivered as evidence develops.

Conclusion

Teenage Pregnancy Strategy: Beyond 2010 sets out a series of strategic aims targeted at preventing conception among those aged under 18 years. These include improving relationships and sex education provision, enhancing access to and use of contraception by young people, and intervening early with those young people who are most at risk of experiencing conception at a young age. It has been argued that in order to demonstrate impact on the outcomes that matter around this issue, strategy and policy and the actions based on such policy need to go beyond good quality information and service provision and take account of the complex interplay of determinants of teenage pregnancy. This includes broader social, cultural and environmental determinants, such as those highlighted by the Marmot Review. These are also very relevant to wider health and wellbeing issues and psychosocial and interpersonal determinants that may benefit from theory and evidence-based activities and approaches to delivery. Of critical importance is the need to evaluate activities that are undertaken to ascertain their efficacy. Without robust evaluation, ineffective approaches taken to address the issue of teenage pregnancy will be unknowingly and expensively repeated, successful approaches will be under-used and under-appreciated, and improvements will rarely be seen.

Discussion questions

- What factors are associated with under-18 conception?
- What public health concerns are associated with under-18 conception?
- What did the Labour Government of 1997–2010 outline as the major facets of their teenage pregnancy strategy?
- Broadly speaking, what does a behavioural change approach involve?

Group-based activity

Consider a typical contraceptive communication event between a health practitioner and a patient (e.g. in a drop-in clinic or GP surgery). Design two potential scripts for how that scenario might play out.

In one, simply provide factual information about contraception and include talk that involves telling the young person what they should do.

In a second, consider asking the young person:

- What they like or don't like about a method of contraception
- What they find easy or difficult about using that method
- What they think other people like them do
- What they think other people want them to do.

Practice role playing the scripts in small groups and see what differences emerge with one person playing the practitioner and one the patient.

Section 2
Fertility and assisted reproductive technologies

Lamiya Mohiyiddeen and Christian Cerra

Introduction

Possibly the single most important risk associated with increasing maternal age is difficulty in conceiving. Fertility declines rapidly with age due to the diminishing number and quality of oocytes and the increased rate of pregnancy loss. Older women are more likely to require reproductive assistance, yet assisted reproductive technologies including *in vitro* fertilisation (IVF) are notably less successful than in younger women. This section covers the effect of aging on fertility and issues surrounding fertility treatment for older women, including underlying concepts, scientific theories and suggested mechanisms, as well as current clinical practice and public policy.

The advent of effective birth control methods, women's increased educational levels and participation in the labour market, and other changes in Western societies over the past century have resulted in a trend to delay childbearing. This has contributed to the growing problem of age-related infertility (Cooke et al, 2011). In the UK, since 2001, births to women aged 35–39 and 40–44 have risen by 1.2% and 2.4%, respectively. This continues the trend of the past two decades; live births to women over 40 have nearly trebled from 9336 in 1989, to 26 976 in 2009 (Office for National Statistics, 2010b). Several epidemiological and demographic studies have shown that increasing female age is linked to decreased fecundity, with a progressive age-related decline in fertility observed from the mid-30s (Menken and Larsen 1986; Leridon 2004). There are multiple factors contributing to this age-related decline in female fertility; a decrease in oocyte numbers and quality hinders the probability of conception with age, together with an increased incidence of early pregnancy loss soon after conception or implantation. Whether assisted reproductive technology (ART) can really compensate for the natural age-related decline in fertility has been a matter of debate. Simulation models of reproduction have shown that even ART cannot make up for the greater than 30–50% loss of fecundity as a result of delayed childbearing. Nevertheless, evidence suggests that for a woman aged 35 years the chances of having a healthy baby are half that of a woman aged 25 years (European Society of Human Reproduction and Embryology Capri Workshop Group, 2005).

Even with the use of IVF technology, both the implantation rate per embryo (van Kooij et al, 1996) and the pregnancy and live birth rate decline markedly in the second half of the third decade (Fécondation In Vitro National, 1995). In a British study of more than 35 000 IVF cycles, maternal age was the most prominent factor in determining chances of success (Templeton et al, 1996). The overall live birth rate per cycle of treatment was the highest among 25 to 30-year-olds; lower rates were observed in younger women (less than 25 years of age) and there was a sharp decrease in older women. In women over 30 years of age, using donor eggs increases the chances of a live birth significantly, but even in the group using donor eggs the chances continue to decrease significantly with age. After adjustment for age, the longer the duration of infertility, the lower the chances of success and live birth rates. Chances of treatment success were higher with a previous pregnancy and live birth, and tended to decrease with each IVF treatment cycle (Templeton et al, 1996).

A 2004 study using a computer-simulated model of reproduction which takes into account biological parameters dependent on age, such as the monthly probability of conceiving, with the risk of miscarriage, etc., found that normally, 75% of women starting to attempt to conceive from the age of 30 years will achieve a pregnancy and a live baby within one year. At 35 years the proportion declined to 66%, and only 44% of women achieved a live birth within a year by the age of 40. If observed during a longer timeframe of four years, the proportion of women who were successful at conceiving in the above three age groups were 91% at 30 years of age, 84% at 35 years, and 64% at 40 years of age, respectively (Leridon, 2004). Women who delayed trying to conceive from age 30 to 35 years resorting to ART can make up for only half of the births lost as a result (an average of 4.2 live births can be 'rescued' with ART from the 8.5 births that would be lost on average by this group of women during those 5 years). In women who decide to delay trying to conceive from the age of 35 to 40 years, ART can only make up for less than a third of births lost in this group (on average 7.1 births out of the 25.2 births normally lost in this group). From this data we can gather that ART at this stage cannot compensate for all births lost by the natural age-related decline of fertility in women (i.e., if a woman starts trying to conceive at age 35 instead of 30, she would normally miss out on about eight chances of having had a successful pregnancy on average during that period, but even using ART she will still have missed out on four chances of having a baby). Therefore, women should be informed of the possible risks of delaying motherhood. However, if they do decide to delay trying for a baby, the chances of success a few years later remain reasonable using ART (European Society on Human Reproduction and Embryology Capri Workshop Group, 2005).

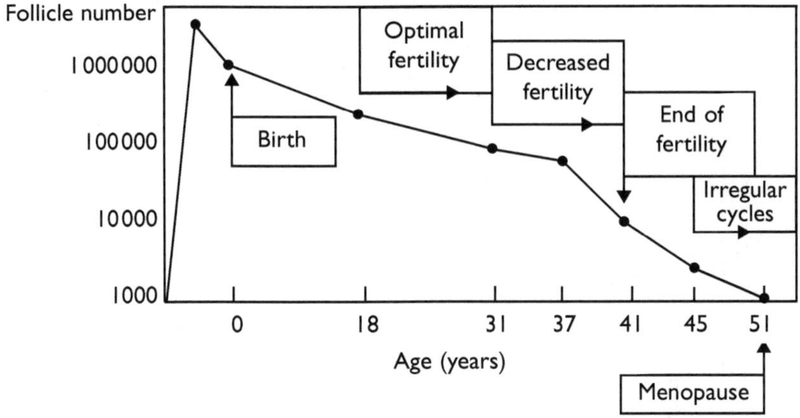

Figure 2.1. The declining oocyte/follicle pool according to Faddy et al (1992) and the corresponding reproductive events (te Velde and Pearson, 2002).

Concepts of reproductive aging

Until a few years ago it was assumed that maternal fertility declined only slightly until the mid-30s. The pattern of ovarian decline was described by Faddy and Gosden as a 'broken stick' whereby an initially linear, slow but steady decline is followed by a sharp acceleration from the age of 37 (*Figure 2.1;* Faddy et al, 1992). Compared to women aged 20 to 24 years, fertility drops by 31% in women aged 35 to 39 years (Menken and Larsen, 1986).

This model is now considered to be outdated, and has been replaced by a pattern of single exponential decline, whereby the rate of decline changes more gradually with the size of the follicle store (*Figure 2.2*; Faddy and Gosden, 1996).

Advanced age and ovarian function

Oocytes derive from germline cells called oogonia, which differ to the cells in the rest of the body (somatic cells) in that they are immortal. Only some of them become primary oocytes, which can begin meiosis (the cell division necessary for the production of more oocytes). When they have entered the first stage of meiosis called Prophase I, they become primary oocytes. In humans, the production of oogonia stops before birth. Oocyte development is halted at this first meiotic division stage until puberty, when levels of gonadotropins rise (ovulation-inducing luteinising hormone, LH) so that the final stages of folliculogenesis

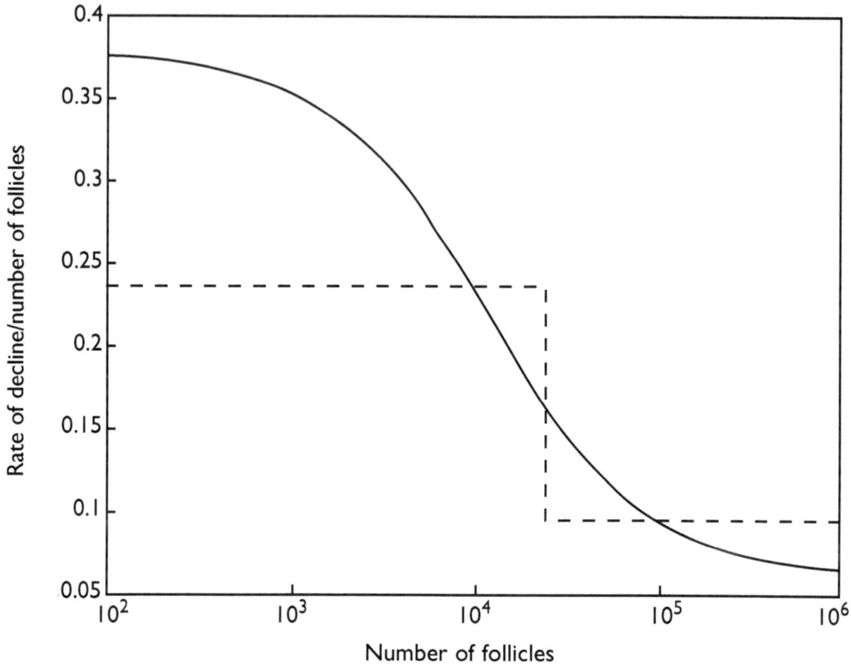

Figure 2.2. Single exponential (gradual) decline model of age-related ovarian decline in the number of follicles versus the previous bi-exponential model (Faddy and Gosden, 1996).

can be achieved (the oocyte becomes a haploid gamete suitable for fertilisation), resulting in ovulation and corpus luteum formation (Peters, 1970). In the fetus, the ovaries have the entire stock of follicles (the oocytes with the surrounding granulosa cells). Only some follicles will reach a selectable phase (antral follicles 2–5mm in diameter). Thereafter, there is an exponential decline in the number of follicles, especially from the age of 37 to 38 onwards. Millions of follicles are present at birth; by puberty only about 300000 are left with hundreds lost undergoing atresia every month, unless rescued by a sudden intercycle rise in follicle-stimulating hormone (FSH), an important factor in early follicular development and survival. Follicles are still lost during anovulatory cycles, pregnancy, breastfeeding and whilst using oral contraceptive methods.

The length of the menstrual cycle is remarkably constant in most women until after the mid-40s. At this time a critical level of a few thousand follicles is reached and the menstrual cycle becomes shorter and irregular due to a shorter follicular phase (Richardson et al, 1987). By the menopause, around the age of 50, the number of follicles is insufficient to sustain the hormonal stimulation necessary for menstruation to occur (Faddy et al, 1992). There is an average period of 10 years between the loss of fecundity (the ability to reproduce) and a definitive arrest of ovarian function. A premature menopause is likely to be associated with an earlier onset of subfertility.

The same factors that influence age at menopause are likely to influence the other reproductive events (such as onset of subfertility, sterility and cycle irregularity). Smoking, for example, is associated with earlier age at menopause, decreased follicular pool, lower natural fertility rate, poorer success rates in IVF, higher FSH levels, and increased incidence of trisomy 21 (Yang et al, 1999). Other factors include severe malnutrition and lifestyle issues.

There is also evidence of a high heritability for age at menopause (around 85% genetically determined, hence the importance of enquiring about family history of early menopause) (de Bruin et al, 2001), highlighting the pivotal role of genetic variation in individual oocyte pool and ovarian aging. Several genes interacting with environmental factors and with other genes may be involved (multifactorial inheritance), including: FSH receptor gene, oestrogen receptor gene, ESR 1, ESR 2, general aging genes (APOE and SOD1), genes involved in apoptosis (programmed cell death) such as BAX1 and BCL2, and also other genes, such as CYP19A1, BMP15, AMH, and AMHR2 (te Velde and Pearson, 2002).

Ovarian reserve markers

As both environmental and genetic factors are involved in the decline of the ovarian pool and oocyte quality, chronological and biological ovarian ages are not equivalent. Assessing biological age is more useful in predicting ART outcomes (Alviggi et al, 2009). Several genetic markers and biomarkers are being developed to help assess biological ovarian aging. ART involves ovarian stimulation using exogenous FSH, which regulates follicular production and maturation in the ovaries by binding to FSH receptor in the granulosa cells. The response to this controlled ovarian stimulation can range from poor response requiring cancellation of the IVF cycle (devastating for the couple) to a dangerously excessive response leading to ovarian hyperstimulation syndrome (OHSS, a complication that can result in oligo-anuria, venous thrombosis, ascites and acute respiratory distress syndrome). It is therefore important to assess the ovarian reserve (the capacity of the ovary to provide eggs that are capable of fertilisation) and the response to FSH stimulation.

Integrative clinical algorithms to assess ovarian aging and predict ovarian response to individualise FSH dosage during fertility treatment are being developed and tested in prospective international trials of biochemical markers of ovarian reserve. So far, basal serum FSH levels (day 2 to day 4 of the menstrual cycle), oestradiol, inhibin B, anti-Müllerian hormone (AMH) levels and antral follicle count (on cycle day 3), have been examined with variable success (Olivennes et al, 2011). Dynamic tests which aim to mimic the response that would be demonstrated to exogenous gonadotropin administration by inducing endogenous FSH release, include clomiphene citrate challenge test (CCCT), gonadotropin analogue stimulation test (GAST) and exogenous FSH ovarian reserve test (EFORT). These tests can also be used as markers of ovarian reserve.

A higher basal serum FSH level, observed from the age of 35 in the early follicular phase, is the first endocrine sign of reproductive aging and predicts a poor response to ovarian stimulation in IVF, with lower chances of conception (Kwee et al, 2003). FSH has an important role in maintaining follicular survival preventing their removal by atresia, and there is a decrease in quality control of the follicles in older women with raised basal FSH levels (te Velde and Pearson, 2002).

Out of all these markers, AMH has the advantage of having relatively stable levels throughout the menstrual cycle and seems to be more specific in assessing ovarian response to gonadotropins, as long as ovarian reserve is reasonably normal and/or patients are not in the extremes of age. AMH is strongly correlated to antral follicle count, and both predictors have a linear relationship with age, reflecting the decline of ovarian reserve with age, although wide individual variation has to be taken into account. In women older than 42 years of age, FSH may have better predictive capacity for ovarian response than AMH. AMH regulates early follicular growth and is secreted by the granulosa cells of antral follicles (Gruijters et al, 2003) as in the case of inhibin B. It is more accurate in providing information on the expected ovarian response to controlled stimulation because, unlike inhibin B, its secretion declines markedly when the follicle reaches the pre-ovulatory phase, therefore reflecting small follicles rather than being confounded by the influence of the dominant follicle (Nardo et al, 2009). However, it is not highly predictive of extremes of responses. Antral follicle count can be performed at the time of baseline ultrasound; however, its interpretation and results are very user dependent. Evaluation of dynamic studies has shown that they are relatively costly and also carry risks associated with hormone therapy.

As shown in a systematic review, all the ovarian reserve markers currently used reflect the number of developing follicles and do not directly reflect the number of primordial follicles or oocyte quality. They also have only limited value in the prediction of extreme responses to stimulation (Broekmans et al, 2006). Information obtained from genetic markers independent of patient characteristics such as age, weight and smoking status may improve the balance between successful outcomes of IVF and the risks of an excessive response to the drugs. In order to optimise outcomes, stimulation protocols could be patient-tailored according to individual variations in the genotype. In particular, FSH receptor gene variants have now been the subject of many studies for their possible role in the response to controlled ovarian stimulation during ART treatment. However, there is still no clear evidence of clinical benefit in the screening for particular genotypes before IVF (Mohiyiddeen and Nardo, 2010).

Poor response to ovarian stimulation during IVF treatment, particularly in women aged 40 years, is a strong predictor of reduced ovarian reserve, which causes a decline in fecundity and early menopause (de Boer et al, 2002; Lawson et al, 2003). Poor response is a stronger predictor of declining ovarian function than raised ovarian reserve markers such as FSH. Age remains the most important factor associated with poor response and embryo quality. A woman older than 41 years and with normal FSH has less chance of conceiving than a woman younger than 41 years showing higher basal FSH levels, even when ARTs are employed (van Rooij et al, 2003). Such evidence supports the concept that age is linked to a rise in aneuploidy and that subfertility is likely to result more from decreased oocyte quality than oocyte numbers.

A study examining how the combined effects of age and FSH affect delivery rates and ART costs required for a live birth found that both age and FSH are important co-predictors of a successful pregnancy. At the highest values of FSH (>12 IU/L) and age (>42 years) tested, these variables dramatically increased the cost of an ART cycle (Henne et al, 2008).

Chromosomal aneuploidy and oocyte quality

It is well known that higher maternal age is associated with a higher incidence of Down's syndrome (detected in 2% of clinical pregnancies among women aged 25 years, and in nearly 35% among women aged 40 years) (European Society on Human Reproduction and Embryology Capri Workshop Group, 2005).

As a result of widespread delay in childbearing age, the incidence has not decreased despite improved antenatal screening. Aneuploidy results in the presence of an abnormal number of chromosomes. This is linked to oocyte quality, as the addition/loss of chromosomes usually occurs during meiosis. Embryos from older women are more likely to show aneuploidy, which contributes to their decline in fecundity by increasing loss of both implantation and early pregnancy. The majority of embryos in women approaching 40 years of age tend to show chromosomal abnormalities.

Oocyte quality is largely determined by genetics, and errors in factors such as oocyte maturation, cell spindle formation, energy supply (for example, deficiencies in mitochondrial proteins) and epigenetics (factors in gene expression that do not involve alterations in the DNA sequence itself, for example, environmental factors can regulate gene expression and imprint on genes which can be passed on), all of which are more likely to occur at an older age.

An oocyte must be able to complete meiosis and mature following appropriate LH stimulation (mid-cycle LH peak), undergo fertilisation and activation, and then coordinate the transcription of gene products for embryonic development, through a complex process involving the cytoskeleton, and genetic and epigenetic mechanisms. An error at any stage of this process may lead to chromosomal abnormalities. Inefficient checkpoints allowing cell cycle progression, despite the presence of errors, may be responsible for aneuploidy.

Oocyte donation

Patients with abnormal or absent oocytes such as those with Turner syndrome and gonadal dysgenesis, as well as women with advanced ovarian age can benefit from oocyte donation. The egg donation process consists of two phases: ovarian hyperstimulation and egg retrieval.

In the first phase, donors receive gonadotropin-releasing hormone injections to suppress the release of LH by the pituitary gland, which drives oocyte maturation. This produces an 'artificial menopause' in order to control the timing of oocyte maturation and ovulation. Subsequently, exogenous FSH is administered to stimulate the ovaries to develop multiple mature oocyte follicles. Once the oocytes have matured, a single injection of human chorionic gonadotropin (hCG) is used to trigger ovulation. During oocyte retrieval, mature eggs are removed from the donor through a surgical procedure called transvaginal ultrasound aspiration. The oocytes are now ready to be fertilised using IVF or intracytoplasmic sperm injection (ICSI) before embryo transfer.

Since the first successful use of donated oocytes in 1984, oocyte donation is often employed during fertility treatment, resulting in good pregnancy outcomes. More than 50% of the women receiving fresh donor eggs are aged over 40. However, according to the Human Fertilisation and Embryology Authority (HFEA, 2012a), 'There is an average 25–40% success rate for each treatment cycle using donor eggs. This is slightly higher than the average success rate for conventional IVF across all age groups, as donor eggs must come from someone aged 35 or under.' Live birth rates for donated eggs are comparable with those for patients' own eggs. The live birth rates for IVF using donated sperm and donated embryos, are also comparable with those couples using their own eggs and sperm (HFEA 2010). Oocytes to be used for fertility treatment are in high demand worldwide as more infertile couples choose this treatment option.

There are distinct groups of oocyte donors; 'patient donors' (women who agree with the fertility clinic to provide a proportion of their own oocytes to 'share' with other women in order to help cover the cost of treatment) and 'non-patient donors' who may be known to the couple. Commercial donation is illegal in the UK; donors are only allowed to claim for reasonable expenses or reimbursement for loss of earnings, etc. There is currently a severe shortage of oocyte donors in the UK, which worsened following changes in the law regarding donor anonymity (Purewal and van den Akker, 2009).

In 2005, UK legislation was changed, requiring any donor of gametes or embryos used in the treatment of others to agree to the disclosure of their identity to any offspring reaching the age of 18. Further amendments to legislation are also having an impact on donor recruitment. The HFEA also made changes regarding arrangements for donor compensation (HFEA, 2010) to implement the European Union's 'Tissues and cells directive'. Under this directive, 'donors may receive compensation which is strictly limited to making good the expenses and inconveniences related to the donation' (Article 12(1) of the EU Tissue and Cells Directive 2004). Following the principles of altruistic donation and cost neutrality, the Revised General Directions 0001 by HFEA, which came into force on 1 April 2012, mean that donors should neither profit nor be penalised financially and only receive modest compensation for loss of earnings: centres are allowed to compensate egg donors up to the fixed amount of £750 per cycle of donation, including loss of earnings and expenses (HFEA, 2012b).

Reproductive aging and public health

In the UK, an upper age limit of 39 is suggested for state-funded IVF treatment on the grounds that IVF success rates decrease with age. However, as previously discussed, success rates in the over 40s are higher when younger donated oocytes are used. Accordingly, use of donated oocytes is much more common after the age of 40. However, ethical issues arise surrounding the possibility of coercion and exploitation due to economic necessity. For example, greater acceptance of 'social egg freezing', whereby women freeze their eggs whilst young may become an option to secure their future reproductive ability (Smajdor, 2011). According to the HFEA, an estimated 3.5 million people in the UK (about 1 in every 6 couples) suffer fertility problems of some kind. While most women will get pregnant within two years without using fertility treatment, 45 264 women received treatment in 2010 and there were 12 714 babies born in 2009 as a result of ART (HFEA, 2010).

Despite such impressive figures, the UK falls short of most other European countries in providing adequate access and funding. Indeed, the UK ranks 17th out of 23 European countries for fertility treatment funded by the state. A report by the European Society on Human Reproduction and Embryology showed that in 2003, the UK carried out 633 IVF treatment cycles per million people in the population; this compares to 2031 in Denmark, 1682 in Belgium and 1009 in France (HFEA, 2010). Apart from the obvious inequality in accessing treatment, the main issue highlighted by these figures is the long waiting times for couples, who sometimes have to wait years for an NHS-funded cycle.

In 2004, the National Institute for Health and Clinical Excellence (NICE) published a guideline recommending that the NHS provide three full cycles of IVF to all couples where the woman is aged between 23 and 39 (treatment should start before the woman's 40th birthday) and has an identified cause of infertility or has had unexplained infertility for at least three years. Despite these recommendations, access to NHS-funded fertility treatment still varies considerably across the country. According to the Department of Health (2009), only 30% of primary care trusts in the UK currently provide three cycles of IVF treatment. A 'postcode lottery' is in place, whereby inclusion/exclusion criteria apply based on factors such as age, body mass index, length of relationships, previous children and previous use of private treatment

There are also implications for the rest of society. IVF, by its nature, adds more individuals who will increase the pressure on state resources. Health costs for mothers and their offspring may place a higher burden on society, given the higher rate of obstetric complications in older women, and the higher rate of babies needing neonatal intensive care in this group. Another issue arising is the one of extreme advanced maternal age (postmenopausal pregnancy), and that facilitating childbearing at a much older age may create the potential to leave children orphaned at a young age. This may create potential social burdens; children may subsequently require social care and psychological support. Such complex ethical scenarios may be prevented by establishing an age limit for mothers accessing fertility treatment (Smajdor, 2011).

Conclusions

The increase in childbearing age is a striking societal change occurring over the past few decades that has lead to the increasingly common issue of subfertility. The age-related decline from the mid-30s in oocyte quantity, and more importantly, in oocyte quality, leading to meiotic non-disjunction and therefore aneuploidy and early pregnancy loss (especially in women aged 40 years or more) are the main features of ovarian aging. There is an apparent discrepancy between the continuing endocrine function, which allows the maintenance of a regular ovulatory cycle pattern until the menopause, and the on average 10 years earlier cessation of female fertility. Because the age at menopause is largely dependent on genetic factors, the rate of ovarian aging may also be largely influenced by heritable factors. Furthermore, women who go through pregnancy over the age of 40 are at increased risk of obstetric complications such as gestational diabetes, pre-eclampsia, and instrumental and caesarean deliveries, and their babies are more likely to need intensive care. Therefore, women should be aware that assisted reproductive technologies can only partially compensate for the loss of fecundity which results from delaying conceiving to a later age.

Discussion questions

- What are the effects of reproductive aging on fertility?
- What factors contribute to the age-related decline in fertility?
- To what extent can the assisted reproductive techniques compensate for the natural age-related decline in fertility?
- In women over the age of 35 years of age, what can significantly improve the success of ART/live birth rate?
- How does the probability of pregnancy change with increasing reproductive age?
- What factors contribute towards premature ovarian failure?
- What is the role of ovarian reserve markers in the clinical practice? Which of the currently available ovarian reserve markers are reliable?
- What factors determine oocyte quality?
- What are the legal implications of oocyte donation in the UK?
- What is the impact of reproductive aging on public health?

References

Abraham C, Michie S (2008) A taxonomy of behavior change techniques used in interventions. *Health Psychology* **27**: 379–87

Abraham C, Wight D, Scott S (2002) Encouraging safer-sex behaviours: Development of the SHARE sex education programme. In: Rutter D, Quine L (eds) *Changing health behaviour*. Open University Press, Buckingham

Allen E, Bonell C, Strange V et al (2007) Does the UK Government's teenage pregnancy strategy deal with the correct risk factors? Findings from a secondary analysis of data from a randomised trial of sex education and their implications for policy. *Journal of Epidemiology and Community Health* **61**: 20–27

Allen G (2011) *Early intervention: The next steps– An Independent report to HM Government*. Cabinet Office, London

Alviggi C, Humaidan P, Howles CM, et al (2009) Biological versus chronological ovarian age: Implications for assisted reproductive technology. *Reproductive Biology and Endocrinology* **22**(7): 101

Baker P, Guthrie K, Hutchinson C, Kane R, Wellings K (2007) *Teenage pregnancy and reproductive health: Summary review*. RCOG Press, London

Bartholomew LK, Parcel GS, Kok G, Gottlieb NH (2001) Intervention mapping: A process for developing theory-and-evidence-based health education programs. *Health Education and Behavior* **25**: 545–63

Bartholomew LK, Parcel GS, Kok G, Gottlieb NH (2006) *Planning health promotion programs: An intervention mapping approach (1st edn.)* Jossey Bass, San Francisco, CA

Bartholomew LK, Parcel GS, Kok G, Gottlieb NH, Fernandez ME (2011) *Planning health promotion programs: An intervention mapping approach (3rd edn.)* Jossey-Bass, San Francisco, CA

Bayley J, Brown KE, Wallace LM (2010) *Improving effective use of ordinary and emergency contraception in adolescents: Findings from a longitudinal questionnaire based study*. Report to Bayer HealthCare by SASH, ARC HLI, Coventry University

Bayley J, Brown KE, Wallace LM (2009). *Improving effective use of ordinary and emergency contraception in adolescents: Findings from a questionnaire based study*. British Psychological Society, Division of Health Psychology Conference. Aston University, Birmingham

Bell J, Clisby S, Craig G, Stanley N, Measor L, Petrie S (2004) *Living on the edge: Sexual behaviour and young parenthood in rural and seaside areas. Teenage Pregnancy Unit Research Briefing*. Department of Health and Department for Education and Skills, London

Broekmans FJ, Kwee J, Hendriks DJ, et al (2006) A systematic review of tests predicting ovarian reserve and IVF outcome. *Human Reproduction Update* **12**(6): 685–718

Brooks F, Morgan A, Magnussen J, Spencer N, Klemera E (2011) WHO Health Behaviour in School Aged Children Study (HBSC) *National Report for England*

2010. Presentation of findings at the Association for Young People's Health (AYPH) Conference. Available from: http://www.youngpeopleshealth.org.uk/tier.aspx?id=2#59

Brown KE, Hurst K, Arden MA (2011) Improving adolescent contraceptive use: Evaluation of a theory-driven classroom-based intervention. *Psychology Health and Medicine* **16**(2): 141–55

Chen X, Wen SW, Fleming N, Demissie K, Rhoads G, Walker M (2007) Teenage pregnancy and adverse birth outcomes: A large population based retrospective cohort study. *International Journal of Epidemiology* **36**: 368–73

Coleman J, Brooks F (2009). *Key data on adolescence. Young people in Brighton.* Available from: www.youngpeopleinfocus.org.uk

Conner M, Norman P (2005) Predicting health behaviour: A social cognition approach. In Conner M, Norman P (eds) *Predicting health behaviour.* Open University Press, Maidenhead

Cooke A, Mills T, Lavender T (2011) Advanced maternal age: Delayed childbearing is rarely a conscious choice. A qualitative study of women's views and experiences. *International Journal of Nursing Studies* **49**(1): 30–9

de Boer EJ, den Tonkelaar I, te Velde ER, et al (2002) A low number of retrieved oocytes at in vitro fertilization treatment is predictive of early menopause. *Fertility and Sterility* **77**(5): 978–85

de Bruin JP, Bovenhuis H, van Noord PA, et al (2001) The role of genetic factors in age at natural menopause. *Human Reproduction* **16**(9): 2014–8

Department for Education and Skills (2006) *Teenage pregnancy: Accelerating the strategy to 2010.* Available from: www.teachernet.gov.uk/publications

Department of Health (2009) *Primary Care Trust survey: Provision of IVF in England 2008.* DOH, London

Department of Health and Department for Children, Schools and Families (2010) *Teenage pregnancy strategy: Beyond 2010.* Department of Health and Department of Children, Schools and Families, London

Department of Health and Department of Children, Schools and Families (2009) *Teenage pregnancy and sexual health marketing strategy.* Department of Health and Department of Children, Schools and Families, London

Department of Health (2011) *Improving behaviour, changing outcomes: A new social marketing strategy for public health.* Department of Health, London

European Society on Human Reproduction and Embryology (ESHRE) Capri Workshop Group (2005) Fertility and ageing. *Human Reproduction Update* **11**(3): 261–76

Faddy MJ, Gosden RG, Gougeon A, et al (1992) Accelerated disappearance of ovarian follicles in mid-life: Implications for forecasting menopause. *Human Reproduction* **7**(10): 1342–6

Faddy MJ, Gosden RG (1996) A model conforming the decline in follicle numbers to the age of menopause in women. *Human Reproduction* **11**(7):1484–6

Fécondation In Vitro National (1995) Pregnancies and births resulting from in vitro fertilization: French national registry, analysis of data 1986 to 1990. *Fertility and Sterility* **64**(4): 746–56

Fuller E (2011) *Smoking, drinking and drug use amongst young people in England in 2010.* London: NHS Information Centre for Health and Social Care

Gruijters MJ, Visser JA, Durlinger AL, et al (2003) Anti-Müllerian hormone and its role in ovarian function. *Molecular and Cellular Endocrinology* **211**(1–2): 85–90

Harden A, Brunton G, Fletcher A, Oakley A, Burchett H, Backhans M (2006) *Young people, pregnancy and social exclusion: A systematic synthesis of research evidence to identify effective, appropriate and promising approaches for prevention and support.* EPPI-Centre, Social Science Research Unit, Institute of Education, University of London, London

Health Development Agency (2003) *HDA delivery plan 2003–2006.* Health Development Agency, London. Available from: http://www.phn-bradford.nhs.uk/NR/rdonlyres/2FDA1E8E-72FE-43B4-8A1C-DD585A78797D/0/HDADeliveryPlan.pdf

Henne MB, Stegmann BJ, Neithardt AB, et al (2008) The combined effect of age and basal follicle-stimulating hormone on the cost of a live birth at assisted reproductive technology. *Fertility and Sterility* **89**(1): 104–10

HFEA (2010) *Fertility facts and figures 2008.* Available from: http://www.hfea.gov.uk/docs/2010_8_Fertility_Facts_and_Figures_2008_Publication_PDF.PDF. [Accessed 13 April 2012]

HFEA (2012a) *Using donated eggs in your treatment.* Available from: http://www.hfea.gov.uk/80.html

HFEA (2012b) *Directions given under the Human Fertilisation and Embryology Act 1990 as amended.* Available from: http://www.hfea.gov.uk/docs/2011-12-21_-_Direction_0001_-_Gamete_and_Embryo_donation.pdf. [Accessed 13 April 2012]

HM Government (2010a) *The Coalition, our programme for government.* Cabinet Office, London

HM Government (2010b) *Healthy lives, healthy people: Our strategy for public health in England.* The Stationary Office, London

HM Government (2011) *Healthy lives, healthy people: Update and way forward.* The Stationary Office, London

House of Lords (2011) *Behaviour change.* The Stationary Office, London

Jayakodi A, Viner R, Curtis K, Sinha S, Roberts H (2005) *Protective and risk factors for early sexual activity and contraception use amongst BME adolescents in East London.* Teenage Pregnancy Unit Research Briefing. Department of Health and Department for Education and Skills, London

Kwee J, Elting MW, Schats R, et al (2003) Comparison of endocrine tests with respect to their predictive value on the outcome of ovarian hyperstimulation in IVF treatment: Results of a prospective randomized study. *Human Reproduction* **18**(7): 1422–7

Lawson R, El-Toukhy T, Kassab A et al (2003) Poor response to ovulation induction is a stronger predictor of early menopause than elevated basal FSH: A life table analysis.

Human Reproduction **18**(3): 527–33

Leridon H (2004) Can assisted reproduction technology compensate for the natural decline in fertility with age? A model assessment. *Human Reproduction* **19**(7): 1548–53

Luker K (2000) *Dubious conceptions: The politics of teenage pregnancy*. Harvard University Press, Cambridge, MA

Marmot M, Allen J, Goldblatt P et al (2010) *Fair society, healthy lives: The Marmot review*. The Marmot Review, UCL, London

Menken J, Larsen U (1986) Fertility rates and aging. In Mastroianni L, Paulsen CA (eds) *Aging, reproduction and the climacteric*. Plenum Press, New York

Mohiyiddeen L, Nardo LG (2010) Single-nucleotide polymorphisms in the FSH receptor gene and ovarian performance: Future role in IVF. *Human Fertility* **13**(2): 72–8

Nardo LG, Gelbaya TA, Wilkinson H et al (2009) Circulating basal anti-Müllerian hormone levels as predictor of ovarian response in women undergoing ovarian stimulation for *in vitro* fertilization. *Fertility and Sterility* **92**(5): 1586–93

National Institute for Clinical Excellence (2004) *Fertility: Assessment and treatment for people with fertility problems*. NICE, London

Newby K (2009) *Under 16 conceptions in the West Midlands: An investigation. Final report for Government Office West Midlands*. Available from: http://www.healthinterventions.co.uk/projects.aspx#project4 [last accessed 4 November, 2011]

Newby K, Bayley J, Wallace LM (2011) "What should we tell the children about relationships and sex?": Development of a program for parents using intervention mapping. *Health Promotion Practice* **12**(2): 209–28

Newby K, Bayley J, Brady G, Sewell A (2011) *Exploring the aspirations of young people at risk of teenage pregnancy: Findings and recommendations*. Coventry City Council, Coventry

NHS Information Centre (2010) *Sexual health statistics for England and Wales 2009*. NHS Information Centre, London

Office for National Statistics (2010a) *Press release, November 23: Conception statistics, England and Wales, 2008*. Available from: http://www.ons.gov.uk/ons/rel/vsob1/conception-statistics--england-and-wales/2008/index.html [Accessed 3 November 2011]

Office for National Statistics (2010b) *Live births*. Available from: http://www.ons.gov.uk/ons/rel/vsob1/characteristics-of-birth-2--england-and-wales/2010/stb-characteristics-of-birth.html [Accessed 13 April 2012]

Office for National Statistics (2012) *Under-18 and under-16 conception statistics*. Available from: http://www.education.gov.uk/childrenandyoungpeople/healthandwellbeing/teenagepregnancy/a0064898/under-18-and-under-16-conception-statistics

Olivennes F, Howles CM, Borini A et al (2011) Individualizing FSH dose for assisted reproduction using a novel algorithm: The CONSORT study. *Reproductive Biomedicine Online* **22**(1): 73–82

Oringanje C, Meremikwu MM, Eko H, Esu E, Meremikwu A, Ehiri JE (2009) Interventions for preventing unintended pregnancies among adolescents. *Cochrane Database of*

Sytematic Reviews, London

Peters H (1970) Migration of gonocytes into the mammalian gonad and their differentiation. *Philosophical Transaction of the Royal Society of London. Series B, Biological Science* **259**(828): 91–101

Purewal S, van den Akker OB (2009) Systematic review of oocyte donation: Investigating attitudes, motivations and experiences. *Human Reproduction Update* **15**(5): 499–515

Reyna V, Farley F (2006) Risk and rationality in adolescent decision making: Implications for theory, practice and public policy. *Psychological Science in the Public Interest* **7**: 1–44

Richardson SJ, Senikas, V, Nelson, JF (1987) Follicular depletion during the menopausal transition: Evidence for accelerated loss and ultimate exhaustion. *Journal of Clinical Endocrinology and Metabolism* **65**(6): 1231–7

Scott ME, Wildsmith E, Welti K, Ryan S, Schelar E, Steward-Streng NR (2011) Risky adolescent sexual behaviours and reproductive health in young adulthood. *Perspectives on Sexual and Reproductive Health* **43**(2): 110–18

Smajdor A (2011) The ethics of IVF over 40. *Maturitas* **69**(1): 37–40

Social Exclusion Unit (1999) *Teenage pregnancy*. Presented to Parliament by the Prime Minister by command of Her Majesty. The Stationery Office, London

Steinberg L (2008) A social neuroscience perspective on adolescent risk taking. *Science Direct Developmental Review* **28**: 78–106

Templeton A, Morris JK, Parslow W (1996) Factors that affect outcome of in-vitro fertilisation treatment. *Lancet* **348**(9039): 1402–6

Te Velde ER, Pearson PL (2002) The variability of female reproductive ageing. *Human Reproduction Update* **8**(2): 141–54

Thaler RH, Sunstein CR (2008) *Nudge: Improving decisions about health, wealth and happiness*. Yale University Press, London

UK Youth Parliament (2007) *SRE: Are you getting it?* Available from: http://www.ukyouthparliament.org.uk/campaigns/sre/AreYouGettingIt.pdf [Retrieved 7 May 2011]

van Kooij RJ, Looman CW, Habbema JD, et al (1996) Age-dependent decrease in embryo implantation rate after in vitro fertilization. *Fertility and Sterility* **66**(5): 769–75

van Rooij IA, Bancsi LF, Broekmans FJ, et al (2003) Women older than 40 years of age and those with elevated follicle-stimulating hormone levels differ in poor response rate and embryo quality in in vitro fertilization. *Fertility and Sterility* **79**(3): 482–8

Viner R, Barker M (2005) Young people's health: The need for action. *British Medical Journal* **330**: 901–3

Wellings K, Kane R (1999) Trends in teenage pregnancy in England and Wales: How can we explain them? *Journal of the Royal Society of Medicine* **92**: 277–82

Yang Q, Sherman SL, Hassold TJ et al (1999) Risk factors for trisomy 21: Maternal cigarette smoking and oral contraceptive use in a population-based case-control study. *Genetics in Medicine* **1**(3): 80–8

Chapter 3

Maternal age and pregnancy risks

Introduction

This chapter presents an in-depth analysis of the evidence surrounding maternal and fetal risks associated with pregnancy and birth in teenagers and older women. Current research is examined to highlight common pregnancy complications and factors that underlie the increase in poor outcomes associated with pregnancy in teenagers and women of advanced maternal age. The clinical implications of the evidence presented in the literature are also discussed in detail, with reference to current guidance and best practice.

Section 1
Young pregnancy and pregnancy complications: Why do women under 19 years of age have increased risk of poor outcomes?

Fiona L Mackie, Melissa K Whitworth and Rebecca L Jones

Introduction

The maternal and fetal complications associated with young pregnancy are outlined and some examples of research examining the causes of these are discussed with practice implications in mind.

Pregnancy outcomes in teenage pregnancies

Pregnancy at a younger age is associated with an increased risk of adverse outcomes for both the teenage mother and her infant when compared to the pregnancy outcomes of women of optimal childbearing age (National Collaborating Centre for Women's and Children's Health, 2010). Two undesirable outcomes which have been widely studied in teenage pregnancies are preterm delivery and delivery of infants with reduced birthweight. Numerous prospective and retrospective studies have been performed on a variety of populations in both developing and developed countries. The findings of the key studies are summarised in *Table 3.1*.

Table 3.1. Summary of key prospective and retrospective studies examining the risk of preterm labour and low birthweight in teenage pregnancy

Author	*Country/ ethnicity (majority)*	*Participants' age/number*	*Pregnancy outcome in teenagers compared to pregnant women of optimum childbearing age*	*Main risk factors identified*
Bukulmez and Deren, 2000	Turkey/ Caucasian	15–17 years 18–19 years 20–24 years *n* = 1490	*Increased:* Preterm delivery Very preterm delivery Low birthweight Intrauterine growth restriction (<10th centile) Intrauterine/neonate death	Socioeconomic factors Inadequate prenatal care Parity Previous obstetric problems
Chen et al, 2007	USA/ Caucasian	10–15 years 16–17 years 18–19 years	*Increased:* Very preterm delivery Preterm delivery Very low birthweight	Gynaecological immaturity Abnormal nutrient partitioning Ethnicity

Although there are conflicting findings from these studies in terms of the absolute risk of adverse pregnancy outcomes, the majority of studies agree that teenagers have a higher rate of premature birth and delivery of lower birthweight infants than pregnant adults. There are several potential reasons for the discrepancies in the different studies, including: small study group sizes, differences in the populations studied (e.g. differences in ethnicity, geographic location, age groups into which participants were subdivided, body mass index, parity, smoking status, adequacy of antenatal care and socioeconomic status), and different ways of defining poor outcome. For example, some studies have examined low birthweight (LBW, <2500g), whilst others have used adjusted birthweight centiles, and a variety of definitions for fetal growth restriction (FGR) and small for gestational age (SGA). In addition, the use of different analytical methods, including adjustment for confounding variables, has a major influence on the specific outcomes of each study.

Susceptibility of teenagers to other poor pregnancy outcomes has also been examined. Studies have reported an increased risk of stillbirth, anaemia, chest infections, urinary tract infections, maternal death, pre-eclampsia and pyrexia of unknown origin (Jolly et al, 2000a; Smith and Pell, 2001; Conde-Agudelo et al, 2005). However, teenage pregnancy has been shown to be beneficial in several respects, including a decreased risk of gestational diabetes, breech presentation, post-partum haemorrhage, induction of labour, operative vaginal delivery, and caesarean delivery (Jolly et al, 2000a; Smith and Pell, 2001; Eure et al, 2002; Conde-Agudelo et al, 2005).

Causes of poor pregnancy outcome in teenage pregnancy

The larger research studies have used sophisticated analytical approaches, including logistic or multiple regressions with adjustments for confounding variables (Frisancho et al, 1983, 1984; Satin et al, 1994; Bukulmez and Deren, 2000; Jolly et al, 2000a), or have excluded subgroups of teenagers to control for confounding variables (Fraser et al, 1995; Chen et al, 2007), in an attempt to delineate the specific factors leading to susceptibility to poor outcome. These have identified a variety of potential influences on poor pregnancy outcome, which can broadly be grouped into biological and behavioural/socioeconomic factors (summarised in *Table 3.2*). Although the majority of these factors are not unique to teenagers, teenagers who become pregnant are more likely to experience them than the general adult obstetric population.

Table 3.2: Summary of potential risk factors for poor obstetric outcome in teenage pregnancy

Biological immaturity	*Demographic/behavioural*
Gynaecological immaturity	Smoking
Skeletal growth	Low socioeconomic status
	Poor nutritional status
	Low gestational weight gain
	Non-attendance at antenatal appointments
	Low educational level
	Black ethnicity
	Parity

Low socioeconomic status

Low socioeconomic status is associated with poor pregnancy outcome in all maternal age groups (Fraser et al, 1995, Bukulmez and Deren, 2000). It is also linked to poor attendance at antenatal appointments, a low educational level, smoking, and poor nutritional status. Unfortunately, delayed booking for antenatal care, low attendance at antenatal clinics and concealed pregnancies are common in teenagers, meaning they may not receive early antenatal advice. Pregnancy is a social stigma for teenagers in some societies, thus psychosocial factors, which may result in stress and/or inadequate social support, may contribute to poor pregnancy outcome (Igwegbe and Udigwe, 2001).

Parity

Parity can influence pregnancy outcome in contrasting ways. Primiparous women are at higher risk of pre-eclampsia and have a tendency to deliver lower birthweight babies than multiparous women. However, several studies show the highest risk of SGA birth is in multiparous teenagers (Smith and Pell, 2001, Khashan et al, 2010). This may be due to a relatively short interpregnancy interval, which is a known risk factor for low birthweight and preterm labour (Zhu et al, 1999). This risk is likely to be related to depleted nutritional stores that have not been sufficiently replenished between pregnancies.

Smoking

All pregnant women, irrespective of age, are advised to stop smoking during pregnancy as there is a wealth of evidence demonstrating that maternal smoking is associated with poor pregnancy outcome, including preterm rupture of the membranes, premature delivery, reduced birthweight, intrauterine growth restriction, placental abruption and sudden infant death syndrome (Andres and Day, 2000). Both nicotine and carbon monoxide, major components of tobacco smoke, are able to cross the placenta and enter the fetal circulation. Nicotine is metabolised into cotinine. Cotinine causes decreased uterine artery blood flow and changes in umbilical artery blood flow which result in altered fetal oxygenation and acid-base balance, and also a decrease in fetal heart rate (Lambers and Clark, 1996). Carbon monoxide also reduces fetal oxygenation. Smoking is a particular problem in teenagers with the reported rate of smoking during teenage pregnancy varying between 19.5% and 50% (Cornelius et al,

2007). In the About Teenage Eating (ATE) study, 50% of teenagers smoked at some stage of their pregnancy; one third quit during pregnancy, leaving a substantial number of teenagers who smoked throughout their pregnancy (Baker et al, 2009). Smoking teenagers had an almost four-fold greater risk of delivering an SGA baby than non-smoking teenagers.

Gynaecological immaturity

Gynaecological immaturity has been highlighted as a major contributor to adverse outcomes in teenage pregnancy, including both preterm labour and low birthweight, particularly in those studies including younger teenagers (aged under 15 years). A low gynaecological age is defined as conception within 2 years of menarche. It is thought that the blood supply to the uterus and cervix may not have had sufficient time to mature, thus the teenagers have a higher risk of sub-clinical infections which are associated with preterm labour (Chen et al, 2007). However, a number of the studies that cite gynaecological immaturity as a cause were unable to record socioeconomic status (Jolly et al, 2000a; Chen et al, 2007), or are not applicable to populations of a 21st century developed country (Frisancho et al, 1983; Conde-Agudelo et al, 2005).

Maternal growth

A major focus of research has been maternal growth in teenage pregnancies. Several prospective studies have investigated whether teenage mothers who are still growing have poor pregnancy outcome due to competition for nutrients with the developing baby. The majority of these studies were performed between the 1980s and the 1990s on predominantly Black and Hispanic pregnant teenagers living in Camden, New Jersey, USA (Scholl et al, 1990, 1994; Lenders et al, 2000). Maternal growth was assessed during pregnancy by measurement of knee-height (from heel to suprapatella) at two time points in pregnancy; an increase in knee-height represents continued long bone growth. These studies found that teenagers who continued to grow whilst pregnant delivered babies that typically weighed less than an equivalent group of non-growing teenagers (on average 150–200g lower birthweight). Growing teenagers were also more likely to deliver premature babies (Scholl et al, 1990, 1994; Hediger et al, 1997). This suggests that in the competition for nutrients, the mother's body wins and so nutrients for growth are preferentially directed to the mother. This is the opposite situation to adult pregnancy, where the baby's needs are always preferentially met (Knopp, 1997). Although the mechanisms underlying this partitioning of nutrients were not examined, the implication was that the normal hormonal and metabolic systems that regulate nutrient availability for the baby are altered when the mother is growing. Since these metabolic changes in pregnancy are induced by the placenta, more recent studies have focused on the role of the placenta in teenage pregnancy.

A recent large prospective study from the UK in 2004 to 2007 (the ATE study), which used a similar method of measuring maternal growth to the Camden, USA study, contradicted the results of Scholl et al. (Baker et al, 2009; Jones et al, 2010). The ATE study found that growing teenagers delivered babies with a higher average birthweight (using customised birthweight centiles) than non-growing teenagers, and delivered more large for gestational age (LGA) infants than non-growing teenagers (Jones et al, 2010). This suggested that the non-growing teenagers were more at risk of SGA birth, indeed, they delivered babies that had a significantly lower birthweight than the normal adult population. The reasons for this are not certain; however, the growing teenagers had a higher average BMI at booking, gained more weight in pregnancy and had a better nutritional status according to their dietary intake of selected micronutrients. This suggests that maternal nutritional status may be a more important determinant of pregnancy outcome in teenage pregnancies. It also implies that teenagers with a poor nutritional status may stop growing themselves, which is a concern in terms of their own development.

There are many potential explanations for the differing results in the Camden and ATE studies. The Camden study found the strongest effects in young multiparous teenagers, whilst the majority of pregnant teenagers in the ATE study were aged 16 to 18 years and in their first pregnancy. The average BMI was higher in the ATE study, in line with current trends of increasing maternal BMI, hence the findings are likely to be more relevant to the majority of the contemporary pregnant teenage population in the UK. Furthermore, the ATE study used adjusted birthweight centiles to define SGA, which has advantages over birthweight alone, particularly in growing teenagers who are more likely to have a small stature.

Poor nutritional status

Poor nutritional status contributes to an increased risk of adverse pregnancy outcomes, especially decreased birthweight and preterm labour (Moran, 2007). Both the quantity and quality of nutrients that the mother consumes are influential.

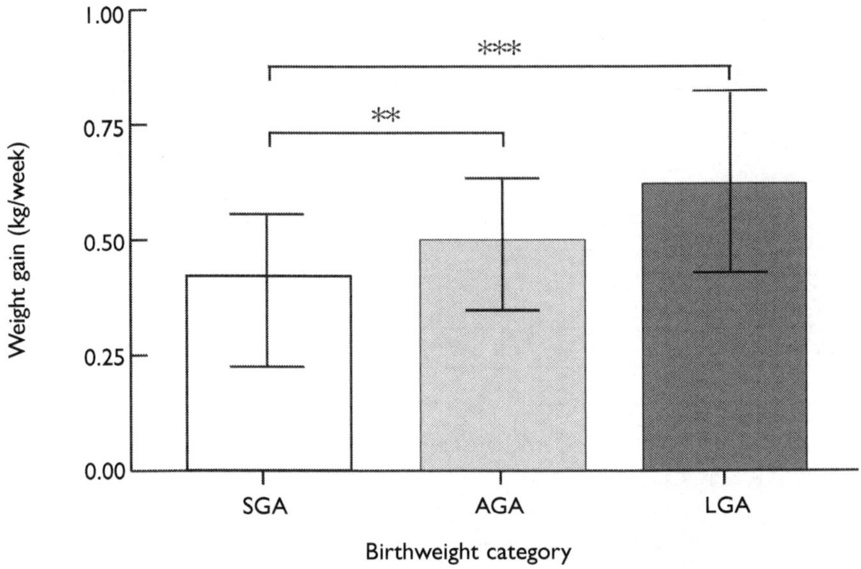

*Figure 3.1. Relationship between gestational weight gain and infant birthweight in teenage pregnancies. Teenagers who deliver SGA infants have a lower gestational weight gain than those who deliver appropriate for gestational age (AGA) infants (**p<0.01) and large for gestational age (LGA) infants (***p<0.001). (Adapted from Jones et al, 2010.)*

Being underweight (i.e. having a BMI <18.5) at the time of entry into antenatal care is an independent risk factor for delivering an SGA infant (Gardosi et al, 1992; Gutierrez and King, 1993). In the ATE study, teenagers who were underweight were more than three times as likely to deliver an SGA baby compared to teenagers who had a normal BMI. Interestingly, teenagers who were obese (BMI >30) at booking also had an increased risk of delivering SGA babies, suggesting they too may be a high risk group. This is consistent with recent findings from adult populations (Gardosi et al, 2009).

Low maternal weight gain during pregnancy is also linked to reduced birthweight and this occurs in teenagers as well (Hediger et al, 1989; Gutierrez and King, 1993; Baker et al, 2009). The ATE study found that teenagers who delivered SGA infants gained less weight during pregnancy than those who delivered normal weight babies (*Figure 3.1*), suggesting that gestational weight gain does play a role in pregnancy outcome in teenagers (Jones et al, 2010). However, the optimal gestational weight gain for teenagers is not currently known

Table 3.3 Institute of Medicine recommendations for total and rate of weight gain during pregnancy, according to pre-pregnancy BMI. Calculations assume a 0.5–2kg weight gain in the first trimester		
Pre-pregnancy BMI (kg/m^2)	*Range of total weight gain (kg)*	*Mean rate and range of weight gain in 2nd and 3rd trimester (kg/week)*
Underweight (<18.5)	12.5–18.0	0.5 (0.4–0.6)
Normal weight (18.5–24.9)	11.5–16.0	0.4 (0.4–0.5)
Overweight (25.0–29.9)	7.0–11.5	0.3 (0.2–0.3)
Obese (≥30.0)	5.0–9.0	0.2 (0.2–0.3)
		(Adapted from Institute of Medicine, 2009)

and no guidance specifically for teenagers has been produced. Pregnant women in the UK are also not routinely weighed after the initial booking appointment as the National Institute for Health and Clinical Excellence (NICE) in England and Wales states that there is insufficient evidence to support its use (National Collaborating Centre for Women's and Children's Health, 2010). The only guidance on ideal weight gain in pregnancy is from the USA Institute of Medicine (IOM) (2009) (*Table 3.3*).

Although adequate macronutrient intake (e.g. protein, carbohydrate and fat) is fundamental to a successful pregnancy, adequate levels of certain micronutrients (vitamins and minerals) are also important. There is a wide range of micronutrients that interact and influence each other. It is believed that there is not a single key micronutrient required for successful pregnancy, but rather a combination (Fall et al, 2003). Although no detailed dietary guidelines exist for pregnancy, several micronutrients are consistently found to be low in the diets of pregnant women, especially pregnant adolescents. Some of these, particularly iron, folate and vitamin A, are known to be important for fetal growth. Teenagers are more prone to having a poor diet, with an abundance of saturated fat, salt and sugar, and a scarcity of fruit and vegetables (Cavadini et al, 2000; Derbyshire, 2009). As well as low dietary intakes of micronutrients, use of vitamin supplements is also low and erratic in teenagers (Stang et al, 2000). There is, however, no good evidence that supplementation with vitamins, including B6, C, D and E or magnesium or zinc has a positive effect on pregnancy outcome (Makrides and Crowther, 2001; Rumbold and Crowther, 2005a, b; Thaver et al, 2006; Mahomed et al, 2007; Ansary et al, 2010).

Often, pregnant teenagers want to improve their diet, and pregnancy is a great driver for change in various health arenas (Burchett and Seely, 2003; National Collaborating Centre for Women's and Children's Health, 2008). However, there are a number of biopsychosocial factors that are implicated in teenagers' dietary habits which may prevent them from making a positive impact on their dietary intake (Burchett and Seely, 2003; Nielsen et al, 2006). These include the influence of peers and family members who may do the food shopping and cooking and not provide the teenager with the opportunity to eat more healthily. Some teenagers have an inability to comprehend the consequences of their current diet on their future health, and a greater concern about their body shape and size. A lack of knowledge of how to eat healthily may also play a role, which is one reason why attending antenatal clinic as early as possible is so important as midwives are the most likely people to give teenagers advice regarding healthy eating. Another major factor is poverty. An in-depth report into UK pregnant teenagers' diets highlighted that many struggle to eat healthily due to a low income (Burchett and Seely, 2003). A lack of money not only causes pregnant teenagers to buy cheap fillers such as biscuits and soft drinks instead of fruit and vegetables, but may also force some to skip meals.

A review of the literature found dietary intakes of the following micronutrients were repeatedly below the recommended amounts in pregnant teenagers in industrialised countries: iron, folate, magnesium, calcium and vitamin E (Moran, 2007). This was reinforced in the ATE study where dietary intakes of iron, folate, magnesium, vitamin D and vitamin A were below the recommended levels for pregnant adult women (Baker et al, 2009). Further analyses revealed that teenagers with the lowest dietary intake of iron (<7.74mg/day) or the lowest dietary intake of folate (<187μg/day) had an almost four-fold increased risk of delivering an SGA baby. These results infer that adequate levels of iron and folate are essential for fetal growth.

Iron

Iron-deficiency anaemia (IDA) is common in pregnancy with 18% of women in industrialised countries and 56% in developing countries becoming anaemic during pregnancy (World Health Organization, 1992). In pregnant teenagers, the incidence is even higher, as demonstrated in the ATE study, in which 64% of teenagers had IDA in the third trimester (Baker et al, 2009). The incidence of IDA in the general population is highest among 15 to 19-year-old girls and if they are already iron-depleted pre-conception, they will be unable to utilise iron stores, which well-nourished women accumulate to sustain fetal growth, especially in late pregnancy (Wahl, 1999; Moran, 2007). Sufficient levels of iron are essential in pregnancy to allow the maternal blood volume to expand adequately, in order to support fetal and placental growth. In addition to increasing the risk of delivering a reduced birthweight infant, a low iron status is associated with maternal and fetal morbidity and mortality, including preterm labour (Allen, 2000). Iron supplementation is beneficial, but iron can be toxic in large quantities and data and advice regarding supplementation is conflicting (Allen, 2000; Rioux and LeBlanc, 2007). A recent publication highlighted that special attention regarding iron supplementation should be paid to adolescents as they have an increased risk of developing IDA (Rioux and LeBlanc, 2007).

Folate

Folate deficiency can cause megaloblastic anaemia, and, in pregnancy, folic acid supplementation has been shown to reduce the incidence of neural tube defects (Mills et al, 1996). The current UK recommendation for folate supplementation is 400µg/day whilst trying to conceive through to 12 weeks of gestation (National Collaborating Centre for Women's and Children's Health, 2008). Despite this advice, only 30% of pregnant women know to use folic acid in the periconception period (Wild et al, 1997). Our recent study investigating folic acid supplementation found lower rates of supplement use in pregnant teenagers than in a comparable pregnant adult cohort. Few teenagers (5%) reported taking pre-conceptional folic acid supplements, due to unplanned pregnancies, and although 70% of pregnant teenagers took supplements in the first trimester, their average duration of supplementation was significantly lower than that of adults (6 vs. 10 weeks) (Jones et al, 2010, unpublished observations).

A low folate status, based either on levels of folate in maternal blood (serum folate) or folate stores (red cell folate) is associated with an increased likelihood of adolescents delivering an SGA baby (*Figure 3.2*) (Baker et al, 2009). However, as demonstrated in *Figure 3.2*, teenagers in the ATE study with a red cell folate concentration above the deficiency threshold, i.e. to the right of the vertical line, still have a raised probability of delivering an SGA infant (approximately 30–35%). This definition of folate deficiency was developed for non-pregnant adults, so their applicability to pregnant teenagers is questionable. These findings provide additional evidence that pregnant teenagers have different nutritional requirements than older women. Low folate status has also been linked to an increased risk of preterm delivery (Scholl et al, 1996).

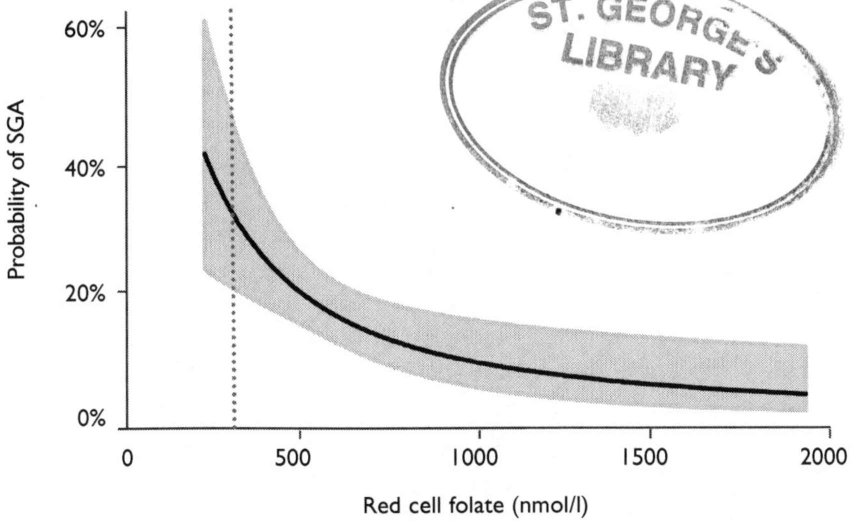

Figure 3.2. Association between maternal folate status in the third trimester and probability of delivering an SGA infant. Teenagers with low red cell folate concentrations have an increased probability of delivering an SGA infant. The vertical line indicates the threshold for folate deficiency at 305nM red cell folate. (Adapted from Baker et al, 2009.)

The placenta in teenage pregnancy

The placenta acts as an interface between mother and baby, and provides the baby with all the nutrients and oxygen needed for growth and survival. It also produces a myriad of hormones necessary for pregnancy and provides a protective barrier for the baby whilst *in utero*. These functions make it vital for a healthy pregnancy.

Little research has been conducted on the placenta in teenage pregnancy. In human pregnancies, the placentas from teenagers who deliver SGA babies are smaller than those who deliver normal weight babies (Hayward et al, 2011b). The growth status of the mother does not appear to have a major impact on placental weight. However, differences in placental function have been detected between adults and teenagers. Amino acids from the mother's blood are an essential nutrient source for the baby. These cross the placenta by specific transporter systems. Studies have found that amino acid transport across the placenta is lower in teenagers than in adults, suggesting placental function is inherently impaired in teenage pregnancy (Hayward et al, 2011a). This may contribute to teenagers' susceptibility to delivering smaller babies. Interestingly, when placentas from growing teenagers were studied, they functioned as efficiently as placentas from adults. This is consistent with growing teenagers delivering higher birthweight infants than non-growing teenagers, as more amino acids will be delivered to promote fetal growth.

Effect of nutritional deficiency on placental development and function

As mentioned previously, poor nutritional status is associated with an increased risk of teenagers delivering SGA infants. This may be related, at least in part, to the effects of important nutrients, such as folate, on the placenta. An ongoing study in Manchester is investigating the effect that folate deficiency in teenagers has on the development and function of the placenta. Pregnant teenagers were recruited in the third trimester and a blood sample taken to assess folate status. Placentas were collected at delivery and placental development and function assessed. Preliminary findings suggest that there are higher levels of cell death in the placentas of teenagers who are deficient in folate in the third trimester of pregnancy (Mackie et al, 2011). This may result in a small or unhealthy placenta that is unable to transfer sufficient nutrients to the baby.

This work offers a potential explanation for the relationship between low folate status and delivery of SGA babies. However, there are still many gaps in our knowledge surrounding why teenagers are at increased risk of poor pregnancy outcome. Overall, the existing studies highlight the challenges of stratifying risk of poor outcome in teenage pregnancies, due to the complex interplay between numerous factors, including growth, parity, age, smoking and nutritional status. As a result, it can be difficult to reduce the risk without broad teenage-focused educational strategies and specialised antenatal care (see *Chapter 4*, Section 1).

Practice implications

There is a huge amount of evidence indicating that teenage pregnancy is associated with poor pregnancy outcome. However, there has been very little research into how to reduce these risks and how best to deliver maternity care to teenagers. NICE recently provided guidelines on service provision for pregnant teenagers, who were recognised as a group whose pregnancies are associated with complex social factors (National Collaborating Centre for Women's and Children's Health, 2010). These recommendations are summarised in *Table 3.4*.

Teenagers perceive a variety of barriers to accessing care. These include: embarrassment of unplanned pregnancy, lack of understanding of the importance

Table 3.4. Summary of NICE recommendations for antenatal services for young women aged under 20 years (Adapted from National Collaborating Centre for Women's and Children's Health, 2010)
Healthcare professionals should: • Offer age-appropriate services • Be aware that the young woman may be dealing with other social problems • Offer information about help with transportation • Offer antenatal care for young women in the community • Provide opportunities for the partner/father of the baby to be involved in the young woman's antenatal care, with her agreement
Commissioners should consider commissioning a specialist antenatal service for young women aged under 20, using a flexible model of care tailored to the needs of the local population. Components may include: • Antenatal care and education in peer groups in a variety of settings • Antenatal education in peer groups offered at the same time as antenatal appointments
Young woman aged under 20 years should be offered a named midwife who should take responsibility for, and provide, the majority of her antenatal care, and provide her with a direct-line telephone number
Healthcare professionals should be given training to ensure they are knowledgeable about safeguarding responsibilities for both young women and their unborn babies
Young women should be offered information that is suitable for their age (including information about care services, antenatal peer group education or drop-in sessions, and housing and other benefits) in a variety of formats

of regular antenatal care, fear of medical procedures and care providers, and concerns regarding confidentiality, age discrepancy, transport problems, financial problems and attitudes of staff. Antenatal services for teenagers must be developed with these barriers in mind and a multidisciplinary/multi-agency approach to care is essential. Whilst no robust research studies have been conducted to demonstrate the direct impact of specialist midwifery or antenatal services on teenage pregnancy outcome, what evidence there is suggests that continuity of care with a specialist service improves engagement (National Collaborating Centre for Women's and Children's Health, 2010).

Many teenagers are reluctant to engage with antenatal services because of fears regarding confidentiality and safeguarding. These fears must be addressed and young people should be made aware of the confidentiality practices and policies of individual maternity services. Local safeguarding guidance must be followed at all times, with safeguarding issues for both the pregnant teenager and the unborn baby being taken into consideration.

Antenatal care must include good dietary advice and assessment of additional needs which may impact on maternal stress levels and ability to eat healthily. Financial and housing needs cannot be overlooked and maternity services must link in with other support agencies both to raise the profile of maternity care and to have a positive impact at an individual level. On average, midwives specialising in teenage pregnancy are in contact with 15 other agencies at any one time, an indication of the complexity of care (Cockerill et al, 2011).

The role that fathers can play in improving pregnancy outcome is often overlooked. Around 25% of fathers of babies born to teenage mothers are aged under 20. Involvement of fathers in antenatal care is essential as they are a key behavioural influence. For example, there is good evidence to show that the strongest influence on maternal smoking is the partner, and providing education for the father on reducing/quitting smoking is essential (Department for Children, Schools and Families, 2008).

Any information provided to pregnant teenagers must be age-specific and tailored to their needs, and parent education should be delivered in an accessible manner. The use of peer educators has been shown to improve acceptability in a number of settings. The development of a peer group can also improve engagement with services. Improving pregnancy outcome in the teenage population requires a multi-faceted flexible approach that takes into consideration a huge number of individual factors and engages the young person within the maternity service and beyond.

Discussion questions

- What complications are teenagers at increased risk of during pregnancy?
- What are the causes of poor pregnancy outcome in teenage pregnancy?
- What barriers to accessing antenatal care do teenagers perceive?
- How can these barriers be overcome?
- How can healthcare professionals improve teenagers' engagement with antenatal services?
- What barriers do individual practitioners face in attempting to offer optimal care to teenagers?
- How can these barriers be overcome?

Section 2
Obstetric risks associated with advanced maternal age

Lucy Higgins and Alexander E P Heazell

Introduction

Advanced maternal age (AMA) is defined by the Royal College of Obstetricians and Gynaecologists (RCOG) as women embarking upon pregnancy at 35 years of age or more (Bewley and Nikolaou, 2009). Mothers of AMA are a heterogeneous population comprising those who have delayed first childbearing, those who have experienced subfertility and those who have continued childbearing. First pregnancies and births are widely accepted to be riskier than subsequent pregnancies, with a higher incidence of stillbirth (Raymond et al, 1994) and hypoxic ischaemic encephalopathy (Mahony et al, 2009). The rising incidence of co-morbidities, particularly obesity, in the AMA population is thought to generate a suboptimal uterine environment for implantation, fetal growth and maternal adaptation to pregnancy, and introduces difficulties in establishing what adverse effects are due to the process of maternal aging alone.

Whilst the incidences of pregnancies and births to women of AMA are increasing, older mothers constitute a relatively small proportion of the obstetric population, accounting for 48 658 births (13%) in a British cohort of 385 120 births between 1988 and 1997 (Jolly et al, 2000b) and a similar proportion of Scottish births in 2005 (*Figure 3.3*) (Smith et al, 2008). The evidence base for clinical practice relating to AMA is sparse, and is largely not of optimal quality (category II or III evidence), usually being drawn from retrospective studies and birth registers. Such data sources may be biased by under-reporting of pregnancies in this age group, particularly those resulting in miscarriage or termination. In addition, they are also incapable of providing background information relating to the reasons for childbearing at AMA, the background socioeconomic and health status of the mother and the influence of paternal age upon pregnancy outcomes. Furthermore, published studies have also employed a variety of age ranges to define both AMA (>35 years, >40 years or >45 years) and control (20–25 years, 20–30 years, <35 years) groups for comparison, reflecting the lack of convincing evidence base for any particular age lying at a consistent threshold for increased risk. Observational studies are also intrinsically confounded by clinicians' preconceived ideas of risk and appropriate management in mothers of AMA; some may adopt lower thresholds for intervention (Roos et al, 2010), particularly

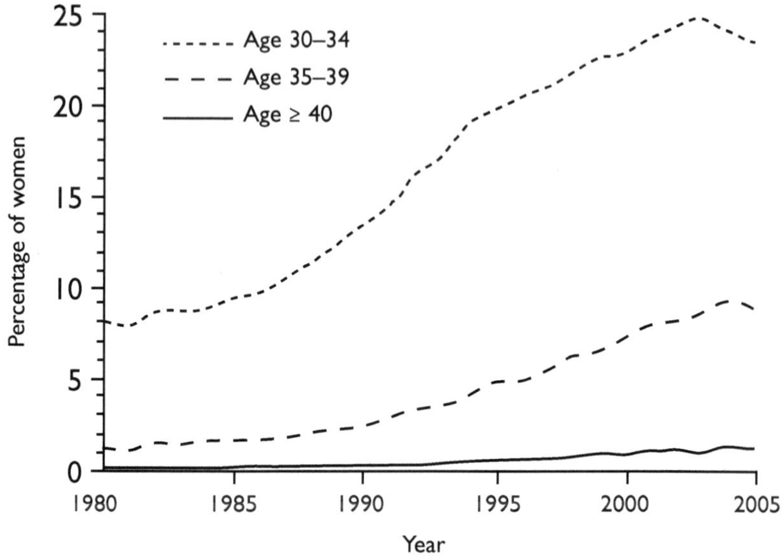

Figure 3.3. Trends in the incidence of pregnancies and births to mothers of advanced maternal age between 1980 and 2005 (Smith et al, 2008).

in primigravidas, whilst others may adopt a less interventional approach, especially in multiparous women. Compared with teenage pregnancy, pregnancy at AMA is less well recognised as a high risk pregnancy and the evidence base to support management of AMA pregnancies is not as strong.

Current guidance from the RCOG recommends that women commence childbearing between the ages of 20 and 29 years and complete their families by 35 years of age (Bewley and Nikolaou, 2009). However, the level of risk acceptable to each individual is intricately linked to that particular woman's reasons for delaying or continuing childbearing, her individual health and social circumstances, and her desire for a child. This highlights the need for excellent preconception care and appropriate family planning advice.

Preconception care

With advancing maternal age the number and quality of oocytes declines sharply and as such, female fertility also declines. The average time to conception is increased beyond the age of 35, and these women are more likely to require assisted reproductive technologies (ART) ranging from ovulation induction to *in vitro* fertilisation techniques with or without the use of donor oocytes (Liu and Case, 2011). Many primary care trusts limit NHS-funded ART to women of less than 40 years of age due to the poor rates of live birth per cycle of treatment at 40 years and beyond (6% compared with 20% at 20–35 years) (National Collaborating Centre for Women's and Children's Health, 2004). Pregnancy following ART is known to be associated with an increased incidence (independent of maternal age and parity) of pregnancy-induced hypertension (Tan et al, 1992), gestational diabetes (Maman et al, 1998), multiple pregnancy (McVeigh, 2007), low birthweight/fetal growth restriction (Wang et al, 1994), and premature delivery (iatrogenic and spontaneous) (Tallo et al, 1995). The use of donor oocytes further increases many of these obstetric risks (Porreco et al, 2005; Henne et al, 2007). Older mothers are also significantly more likely to have significant co-morbidities including obesity, chronic hypertension and diabetes prior to embarking upon pregnancy (Montan, 2007), highlighting the essential need for adequate pre-conception counselling and access to family planning, including termination of pregnancy services, to enable informed reproductive choice.

Early pregnancy complications

Once pregnancy is achieved, there is a significantly increased rate of miscarriage amongst women of AMA from around 11–12% in women aged 20–29 years to 24.6%, 51% and 93.4% at 35–39, 40–44 and ≥45 years, respectively (Nybo et al, 2000). The increased incidence of miscarriage and recurrent miscarriage remains elevated even after exclusion of pregnancies affected by aneuploidy and serious congenital abnormality. This suggests a role for two potential aetiologies; poor quality of the ovum and/or an adverse uterine environment. Interestingly, the potentially life-threatening early pregnancy complication of ectopic pregnancy is observed to increase almost five fold between age 21 (1.4%) and 44 (6.9%) (Nybo et al, 2000); this may be related to tubal blockage (caused by the accumulation of adhesions) or poor tubal motility. Older mothers are also more likely to experience significant bleeding during pregnancy (Yang et al, 2005) including threatened miscarriage and antepartum haemorrhage.

There is a well-documented association of maternal age and fetal aneuploidy, particularly of Down's syndrome (trisomy 21), predominantly due to maternal chromosomal non-disjunction in meiosis. Such pregnancies are more likely to spontaneously miscarry or to be terminated. The risk of giving birth to a child with Down's syndrome escalates from approximately 1 in 1350 at 25 years of age, to 1 in 350 at 35 years, to 1 in 85 at 40 years and further still to 1 in 35 at 45 years of age (Morris et al, 2003). Despite this, due to the relatively low (although increasing) proportion of pregnancies occurring at AMA, and the higher uptake of Down's syndrome testing among these women, more children with Down's syndrome are born to women under the age of 35 than in any other age group. There is, however, a less well-recognised association of advanced maternal age with non-chromosomal fetal anomaly. Cleary-Goldman et al (2005) observed adjusted odds ratios for congenital anomalies of 1.4 and 1.7 for women aged 35 to 39 and ≥40 years of age, when compared to mothers aged <35 years. A range of fetal anomalies have been linked with reproductive aging, independent of co-morbidities and use of pharmaceutical drugs. These include cardiac defects (odds ratio 1.2; 95% CI 1.03–1.22), hypospadias (odds ratio 1.85; 95% CI 1.33–2.58), other male genital tract abnormalities (odds ratio 1.25; 95% CI 1.08–1.45) and craniosynostosis (odds ratio 1.65; 95% CI 1.18–2.30) (Reefhuis and Honein, 2004). The described abnormalities are of varying degrees of consequence for the offspring, from miscarriage and stillbirth to survival with or without disability. The causes of such abnormalities are incompletely understood with suggested mechanisms including poor ovum quality, multiple pregnancies and use of ART.

Whether spontaneous or assisted, multiple pregnancy is recognised to occur more frequently in association with advancing maternal age with reported incidences of 1.4% between 20 and 34 years of age, rising to 4.1% and 5% between 30–39 and 40–49 years of age, respectively, and escalating to 37% at the age of 50 or more (Salihu et al, 2003). Spontaneous multiple pregnancies are thought to occur due to increased follicle-stimulating hormone levels during the follicular phase of the menstrual cycle, resulting in the maturation of two or more co-dominant follicles and thus in dizygotic twinning. Whilst women who have experienced primary infertility may view twin pregnancy as a positive opportunity to both start and complete their family, multiple pregnancy is associated with a greatly increased rate of (potentially life-threatening) maternal and fetal pregnancy complications, including pre-eclampsia and non-proteinuric pregnancy-induced hypertension, gestational diabetes, anaemia, placenta praevia, caesarean section, postpartum haemorrhage, miscarriage, fetal abnormality, fetal death *in utero*, neurodevelopmental impairment and FGR (Braude, 2006). The Human Fertilisation and Embryology Authority (HFEA) and the RCOG are currently promoting the use of single embryo transfer to reduce risks of multiple pregnancy in those most at risk (McVeigh, 2007).

Late pregnancy complications

Perhaps unsurprisingly, given the increased incidence of chronic hypertension with advancing age, there is an increased incidence of pregnancy-induced hypertension and pre-eclampsia in older mothers (Vigil-De Gracia et al, 2004). The risk of superimposed pre-eclampsia is reported to be approximately 10–25% for those with mild chronic hypertension, but as high as 50% for those with severe chronic hypertension (Sibai, 2002). There is also a recognised clustering of other independent risk factors for the development of pre-eclampsia in the AMA population including age ≥40 years at first childbearing, or an inter-pregnancy interval of ≥10 years; obesity; and other co-morbidities, particularly renal disease and diabetes. At the age of 44 years or more, the relative risk of pregnancy-induced hypertension is 2.8 (95% CI 2.5–3.1) (Schoen and Rosen, 2009). Such constellations of risk factors may warrant the prescription of 75mg aspirin once daily as pre-eclampsia prophylaxis from 12 weeks' gestation under the guidance of NICE (National Collaborating Centre for Women's and Children's Health, 2011).

AMA is also a recognised risk factor for development of gestational diabetes mellitus (GDM); after the age of 44 years the relative risk of developing GDM is increased by a factor of 11.2–14.2 (Schoen and Rosen, 2009). Even mild degrees of impaired glycaemic control are associated with macrosomia, fetal hyperinsulinaemia, and caesarean delivery (Metzger et al, 2008) and it is known that GDM is a risk factor for the subsequent development of type 2 diabetes mellitus (Kim et al, 2002). Yet despite this known association, maternal age is currently absent from the list of criteria to screen for GDM (National Collaborating Centre for Women's and Children's Health, 2008a). The rationale provided for this omission is the lack of convincing data that this would be of economic benefit (National Collaborating Centre for Women's and Children's Health, 2008a). As evidence accumulates, it is anticipated that universal screening for GDM will eventually be adopted.

Independent of other pregnancy complications, maternal age is independently associated with an increased risk of fetal growth restriction (Montan, 2007), a recognised contributor to over 50% of all stillbirths (Gardosi et al, 2005) and a principal cause of iatrogenic premature delivery. Fetal growth restriction is principally of placental origin, raising further questions about the importance of oocyte quality and of the interaction between the placenta and the uterus. Further evidence for impaired control of placental implantation in mothers of AMA is provided by the increased incidence of not only placenta praevia but also morbid placental adherence (Wu et al, 2005), both of which infer a greatly increased risk of obstetric haemorrhage, blood transfusion, peripartum hysterectomy and maternal mortality. In fact, older pregnant women are significantly more likely than their younger counterparts to experience massive obstetric haemorrhage in the context of placenta praevia (Hasegawa et al, 2009). Premature separation of the placenta (placental abruption) is also independently associated with AMA (Sheiner et al, 2003) with disastrous consequences for both mother and fetus.

A new challenge facing maternity services is the increasing prevalence of cancer, both prior to and during pregnancy (Pereg et al, 2008). In particular, the incidence of breast cancer rises sharply from 35 years of age (with a background lifetime risk of 1 in 9 women), and risk is temporarily further increased during the postnatal period (Han et al, 2010). This is compounded by difficulty in detection during the antenatal and postnatal period due to the evolving changes in breast tissue. Improved cancer therapies mean that more women are surviving cancer, and more selective treatments mean that many of these women remain fertile. The effect of pregnancy on the incidence, severity and treatment of cancer recurrence (particularly hormone-sensitive tumours) is not clearly understood (Valachis et al, 2010). In early pregnancy, the diagnosis of cancer in the mother may lead to a decision to terminate in the interests of prompt maternal treatment. In late pregnancy, such diagnosis may prompt iatrogenic preterm delivery to enable maternal treatment. In previable or very preterm gestations the risk–benefit ratio may be considered to support maternal treatment during pregnancy. Surgical treatment of primary cancers may be possible during pregnancy and certain types of chemotherapy (particularly those that are heavily protein bound and therefore unlikely to cross the placenta) may be administered in the second trimester of pregnancy. Radiotherapy to selected organ targets, particularly in low dose, with abdominal shielding in sites distant to the uterus, may be considered appropriate in the management of certain cancers. The woman receiving anticancer therapy during pregnancy requires close fetal surveillance for fetal growth restriction and fetal anomaly (Pentheroudakis and Pavlidis, 2006).

Labour

Mothers of AMA more frequently experience both preterm birth and postmature pregnancy. Preterm birth in particular is a major contributor to perinatal mortality and morbidity and to long-term infant health problems (Saigal and Doyle, 2008). Extreme AMA (≥45 years of age) is also associated with an increased risk of early preterm birth (<34 weeks' gestation) with an odds ratio of 3.5 (95% CI 1.4–9.0), and outcomes of early preterm birth in AMA are poorer than those of younger mothers (Yogev et al, 2010). Whilst many preterm births in women of AMA are iatrogenic due to pregnancy complications or comorbidities (Ip et al, 2010), AMA remains an independent risk factor for spontaneous preterm birth (Carter et al, 2011). In particular, preterm prelabour rupture of membranes precedes 40% of all preterm deliveries (Maxwell, 1993) and occurs more commonly in mothers of AMA compared to younger mothers (Carter et al, 2011). Unfortunately, neonatal outcomes following preterm prelabour rupture of membranes in AMA are poor in comparison to those of younger mothers (Pasquier et al, 2009).

Conversely, pregnancy at AMA is also more likely to be complicated by postmaturity (Roos et al, 2010) which is of particular relevance given the increased rate of stillbirth in the AMA population at term. NICE currently recommends that induction of labour should be offered to all women whose pregnancies remain undelivered after 41 completed weeks of gestation due to relative reduction in risk of a variety of maternal and neonatal outcomes, including perinatal mortality (National Collaborating Centre for Women's and Children's Health, 2008b). No national recommendation has been made regarding earlier elective delivery in mothers of AMA although many practitioners are already doing so. Older women are more likely to undergo induction of labour, but such inductions of labour are also more likely to fail to establish active labour and therefore require caesarean section delivery (Roos et al, 2010).

When labour does establish it is more likely to be dysfunctional and require augmentation with oxytocin analogues (Treacy et al, 2006) or operative vaginal delivery (Wang et al, 1994; Treacy et al, 2006). Overall, it has been observed that the rate of oxytocin augmented labours resulting in caesarean section increases to 7.4% in women aged over 35 years from a baseline of 3.5% in the 20–25 year age group (Treacy et al, 2006). In particular, the rate of failed trial of vaginal birth after caesarean section is increased in mothers of AMA (Eden et al, 2010). The caesarean section rate remains elevated even after exclusion of confounding co-morbidities and variables, including induction of labour (Gilbert et al, 1999; Heffner et al, 2003; Bayrampour and Heaman, 2010). There are few studies that have examined the effect of aging on the structure and function of the uterus. It has been observed that myometrial contractility is linearly reduced with increasing maternal age which may explain the increased rate of dysfunctional labour and interventions to correct this (Smith et al, 2008).

Mothers of AMA are more likely to experience obstetric anal sphincter injury following vaginal delivery than are younger mothers (Hornemann et al, 2010). This excess risk is partly, but not entirely, explained by the increased incidence of risk factors for obstetric anal sphincter injury (such as induction of labour, instrumental delivery and shoulder dystocia) in this population. Whilst the recognition and repair of such injuries is improving, even with optimal care following injury 20–40% of women are troubled with anal incontinence symptoms at 12 months postpartum (Malouf et al, 2000). There is no role for the routine use of episiotomy to prevent obstetric anal sphincter injury (Carroli and Mignini, 2009). Although selective use of right mediolateral episiotomy does reduce its incidence (Eogan et al, 2006), this has not been specifically studied in the AMA population. There is conflicting evidence regarding the effect of pregnancy and delivery at AMA on urinary continence mechanisms (particularly pelvic floor tone) and subsequent urinary incontinence (Hijaz et al, 2012). The benefit of postpartum pelvic floor exercises has not been specifically examined in the AMA population. Shoulder dystocia displays a marginal increase in incidence in mothers of AMA after the exclusion of comorbid risk factors such as diabetes, induction of labour and instrumental delivery (Tsur et al, 2011). Shoulder dystocia is associated with maternal morbidity (including obstetric anal sphincter injury and postpartum haemorrhage) and fetal morbidity (including hypoxic ischaemic encephalopathy and brachial plexus injuries) and mortality. However, prediction and prevention of shoulder dystocia are notoriously inaccurate/ineffective.

Postpartum

Following birth, mothers of AMA are more likely to experience postpartum haemorrhage (Montan, 2007; Shrim et al, 2010; Yogev et al, 2010) compared with their younger counterparts. As uterine atony accounts for approximately 80% of all postpartum haemorrhages, the mechanism underlying increased rates of haemorrhage may be related to reduced myometrial contractility (Smith et al, 2008). As one of the leading causes of maternal mortality in the UK, active management of the third stage of labour for the prevention of postpartum haemorrhage should be offered to all women and the early recognition and effective management of haemorrhage is imperative; this vigilance should be heightened in the care of mothers of AMA, particularly those with additional risk factors for haemorrhage.

Other less common intrapartum complications have been linked to AMA including an increased rate of uterine rupture and amniotic fluid embolism. Uterine rupture occurs more frequently in mothers of AMA than younger mothers, and this risk remains elevated even after adjustment for parity, and induction or augmentation of labour (Zwart et al, 2009). The UK Obstetric Surveillance System (UKOSS) has observed an increase in the rate of amniotic fluid embolism in older women from ethnic minorities (Abenhaim et al, 2008). Once more, prediction and prevention remain largely ineffective.

Emotional health

AMA has not been found to be linked to the diagnosis of postnatal depression (Eastwood et al, 2011). AMA was also unrelated to the incidence of major depressive disorder (background rate 8%) in an Australian prospective cohort study of 592 nulliparous women of whom 189 were aged 37 years or more (McMahon et al, 2011). The reasons for this low rate may be related to the differing socioeconomic and educational statuses of younger and AMA mothers. There is however a documented link between AMA and psychosis (onset within the first 90 days after delivery) in first time mothers without past psychiatric history (Valdimarsdottir et al, 2009). Mothers of AMA with mental health problems should be managed in perinatal mental health networks as described by NICE (National Collaborating Centre for Mental Health, 2007).

Maternal and perinatal mortality

Sequential reports from the Confidential Enquiries into Maternal Deaths have demonstrated that the risk of maternal mortality from both direct and indirect causes in older mothers aged 35–39 and ≥40 years outstrips that of women aged 20–24 and 25–29 years by several fold (*Figure 3.4*), in particular, deaths from cardiac disease which is the leading cause of maternal death (Centre for Maternal and Child Enquiries, 2011). Advanced age is a significant risk factor for venous thromboembolism, which in the penultimate Centre for Maternal and Child Enquiries (CEMACE) report was the primary cause of direct maternal death, decreasing in the last triennia due to raised awareness and guidance concerning risk assessment and thromboprophylaxis. Once more, AMA tends to cluster with other risk factors for thromboembolism such as obesity, smoking and comorbidities, and as such it is essential that regular venous thromboembolism risk assessments are carried out and acted upon, particularly peripartum. The UKOSS is currently monitoring the incidence of a number of maternal pathologies with links to vascular pathology, known to be increased in incidence in older women, particularly in pregnancy and delivery. These conditions include stroke, myocardial infarction, aortic dissection and cardiac arrest (Knight et al, 2011). Peripartum cardiomyopathy is also recognised to be more common in the AMA population, and has a high mortality rate (Abboud et al, 2007).

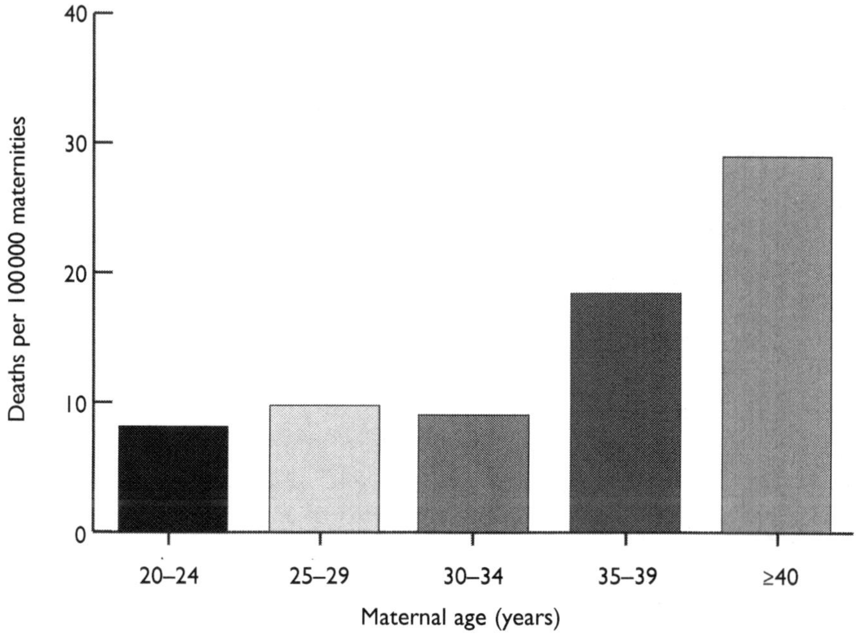

Figure 3.4. Maternal mortality rates by maternal age between 2006 and 2008. (Adapted from Centre for Maternal and Child Enquiries, 2011.)

A systematic review of AMA cohort and case-control trials has demonstrated an increased risk of stillbirth with advancing maternal age (*Figure 3.4*), yet the magnitude of this risk is highly variable (Huang et al, 2008). The risk of stillbirth in relation to maternal age follows a J-shaped curve with the lowest incidence of 4 in 1000 at 25–29 years of age (reflecting the increased number of second or subsequent births in this age group in comparison to births at 20–24 years of age) and a steep incline after the age of 40 years (Carolan and Frankowska, 2011), reaching 8.3 in 1000 at ≥45 years of age (Nybo et al, 2000), although stillbirth was defined in this study as fetal loss beyond 28 completed weeks' gestation. The age-related incidence of fetal loss after 20 weeks' gestation was examined by Reddy et al (2006) who concluded that whilst there was a relative risk of stillbirth in those aged 35–39 and ≥40 years of 1.32 and 1.88, respectively, compared with mothers aged under 35 years, the absolute risk of stillbirth was only 1 in 382 and 1 in 267 for pregnancies in the age ranges 35–39 years and ≥40 years, respectively. The increased risk of stillbirth is observed to persist even after adjustment for confounding variables which include the increased rate of pre-pregnancy and gestational co-morbidities (Jolly et al, 2000b).

There is also a specific increase in the number of stillbirths for which no cause is identified in AMA (Bateman and Simpson, 2006). As the principal determinant of fetal growth and the exchange surface for nutrients and gases, it is hypothesised that placental dysfunction may explain many 'unexplained' stillbirths in AMA. The structure and function of the placenta in maternal aging however remains largely unstudied. The majority of stillbirths in AMA occur in late gestation, with risks accelerating after 39 weeks of pregnancy (Reddy et al, 2006). This knowledge has generated disparate practice worldwide regarding active delivery (induction of labour at term or elective caesarean section) or expectant management of delivery (Roos et al, 2010), often guided by anxieties of the physician or expectant mother, yet the neurodisability burden of elective early term delivery is not to be underestimated (MacKay et al, 2010).

In addition to the recognised increased rates of stillbirth in mothers of AMA, the risks of AMA continue following birth, with neonatal morbidity (Shrim et al, 2010) and death (Jacobsson et al, 2004) being increased in mothers of AMA. The perinatal mortality rate is increased to a relative risk of 2.4 (2.2–2.7) after 44 years of age compared with younger mothers (Schoen and Rosen, 2009); the majority of this increased burden is due to stillbirths.

The benefits of AMA

Socially, there may be many benefits of later childbearing including the completion of further education, career progression and financial stability. It is known that many older mothers who intentionally delay pregnancy are of higher income, educational status and socioeconomic class than those who have their children early. They may also lead healthier lifestyles, attend earlier for antenatal care or pay for private antenatal and intrapartum care which may predispose to increased investigation, diagnosis and interventions (Stein and Susser, 2000; Viau et al, 2002; Loke and Poon, 2011). This will be further discussed in *Chapter 6*, Section 2.

Conclusion

The demographic of the maternity population is changing. Healthcare providers and healthcare systems must adapt rapidly to the increased demands that AMA will place upon resources. It should be recognised that pregnancy at AMA carries an increased risk of both maternal and fetal morbidity and mortality, but that these risks in general remain low. Currently there is insufficient evidence upon which to recommend a particular care pathway; predictive tests for the development of subsequent problems are either non-existent or insufficiently sensitive or specific. There is an urgent need for high quality research to elucidate the mechanisms underlying reproductive pathologies of AMA and their most effective management, with which to create national evidence-based guidelines for the care of older mothers. In the meantime, awareness of the risks of pregnancy at AMA is essential among both healthcare workers and the public, and should be included within healthcare professional teaching and family planning consultations.

Discussion questions

- Are clinicians, and the population in general, adequately informed regarding the risks of pregnancy and childbearing at AMA? What can be done to further this understanding given the widespread inadequacy of pre-pregnancy counselling services in the UK?
- Given the risks of infertility treatment and the low success rate, should treatment be provided (either by the National Health Service or privately funded) for women of advanced, particularly extremely advanced, maternal age? What factors should be considered when making this decision?
- In the absence of quality research upon which to recommend any particular maternity care pathway for women of AMA how can we ensure women receive the best possible pregnancy care? Should all women embarking upon pregnancy over the age of 35 be registered in a national audit, for example by the UK Obstetric Surveillance System?

References

Abboud J, Murad Y, Chen-Scarabelli C, Saravolatz L, Scarabelli TM (2007) Peripartum cardiomyopathy: A comprehensive review. *International Journal of Cardiology* 118(3): 295–303

Abenhaim HA, Azoulay L, Kramer MS, Leduc L (2008) Incidence and risk factors of amniotic fluid embolisms: A population-based study on 3 million births in the United States. *American Journal of Obstetrics and Gynecology* **199**(1): 49 e1–8

Allen LH (2000) Anemia and iron deficiency: Effects on pregnancy outcome. *American Journal of Clinical Nutrition* **71**: 1280S–84S

Andres RL, Day M (2000) Perinatal complications associated with maternal tobacco use. *Seminars in Neonatology* **5**: 231–41

Ansary A, Palacios C, De-Regil L, Pena-Rosas J (2010) Vitamin D supplementation for women during pregnancy. *Cochrane Database of Systematic Reviews* CD008873

Baker PN, Wheeler SJ, Sanders TA, et al (2009) A prospective study of micronutrient status in adolescent pregnancy. *American Journal of Clinical Nutrition* **89**: 1114–24

Bateman BT, Simpson LL (2006) Higher rate of stillbirth at the extremes of reproductive age: A large nationwide sample of deliveries in the United States. *American Journal of Obstetrics Gynecology* **194**(3): 840–5

Bayrampour H, Heaman M (2010) Advanced maternal age and the risk of cesarean birth: A systematic review. *Birth* **37**(3): 219–26

Bewley SLW, Nikolaou, D (2009) *Consensus views arising from the 56th Study Group: Reproductive Ageing*. RCOG Press, London

Braude P (2006) *One child at a time. Reducing multiple births after IVF. Report of the Expert Group on Multiple Births after IVF.* Human Fertilisation and Embryology Authority, London. Available from: http://www.oneatatime.org.uk/images/MBSET_report_Final_Dec_06.pdf [Accessed 9 December 2011]

Bukulmez O, Deren O (2000) Perinatal outcome in adolescent pregnancies: A case-control study from a Turkish university hospital. *European Journal of Obstetrics and Gynecology and Reproductive Biology* **88**: 207–12

Burchett H, Seely A (2003) *Good enough to eat? The diet of pregnant teenagers.* Maternity Alliance/Food Commission, London

Carolan M, Frankowska D (2011) Advanced maternal age and adverse perinatal outcome: A review of the evidence. *Midwifery* **27**(6): 793–801

Carroli G, Mignini L (2009) Episiotomy for vaginal birth. *Cochrane Database of Systematic Reviews* **1**: CD000081

Carter MF, Fowler S, Holden A, Xenakis E, Dudley D (2011) The late preterm birth rate and its association with comorbidities in a population-based study. *American Journal of Perinatology* **28**(9): 703–7

Cavadini C, Siega-Riz AM, Popkin BM (2000) US adolescent food intake trends from 1965 to 1996. *Archives of Diseases of Childhood* **83**: 18–24

Centre for Maternal and Child Enquiries (2011) Saving mothers' lives: Reviewing maternal deaths to make motherhood safer: 2006–2008. *British Journal of of Obstetrics and Gynaecology* **118**(s1): 1–203

Chen X, Wen SW, Fleming N, Demissie K, Rhoads GG, Walker M (2007) Teenage pregnancy and adverse birth outcomes: A large population based retrospective cohort study. *International Journal of Epidemiology* **36**: 368–73

Cleary-Goldman J, Malone FD, Vidaver J, et al (2005) Impact of maternal age on obstetric outcome. *Obstetrics and Gynecology* **105**(5 Pt 1): 983–90

Cockerill R, Patawari S, Bennett G, Whitworth M (2011) Care of pregnant young women aged under 20 – models of service provision in the North West. *Archives of Disease in Childhood - Fetal Neonatal Education* **96**: Fa137

Conde-Agudelo A, Belizn JM, Lammers C (2005) Maternal-perinatal morbidity and mortality associated with adolescent pregnancy in Latin America: Cross-sectional study. *American Journal of Obstetrics and Gynecology* **192**: 342–49

Cornelius MD, Goldschmidt L, DeGenna N, Day N (2007) Smoking during teenage pregnancies. *Nicotine and Tobacco Research* **9**: 739–50

Department for Children, Schools and Families (2008) *Teenage parents: Who cares? A guide to commissioning and delivering maternity services for young parents.* Department for Children, Schools and Families, London

Derbyshire E (2009) Dietary habits of pregnant and non-pregnant adolescents. *Nutrition and Food Science* **39**: 490-98

Eastwood JG, Phung H, Barnett B (2011) Postnatal depression and socio-demographic risk: Factors associated with Edinburgh Depression Scale scores in a metropolitan area of New South Wales, Australia. *Australian and New Zealand Journal of Psychiatry* **45**(12): 1040–6

Eden KB, McDonagh M, Denman MA, et al (2010) New insights on vaginal birth after cesarean: Can it be predicted? *Obstetrics and Gynecology* **116**(4): 967–81

Eogan M, Daly L, O'Connell PR, O'Herlihy C (2006) Does the angle of episiotomy affect the incidence of anal sphincter injury? *British Journal of Obstetrics and Gynaecology* **113**(2): 190–4

Eure CR, Lindsay MK, Graves WL (2002) Risk of adverse pregnancy outcomes in young adolescent parturients in an inner-city hospital. *American Journal of Obstetrics and Gynecology* **186**: 918–920

Fall CH, Yajnik CS, Rao S, Davies AA, Brown N, Farrant HJ (2003) Micronutrients and fetal growth. *Journal of Nutrition* **133**: 1747S–56S

Fraser AM, Brockert JE, Ward RH (1995) Association of young maternal age with adverse reproductive outcomes. *New England Journal of Medicine* **332**: 1113–7

Frisancho AR, Matos J, Bollettino LA (1984) Influence of growth status and placental function on birth weight of infants born to young still-growing teenagers. *American Journal of Clinical Nutrition* **40**: 801–7

Frisancho AR, Matos J, Flegel P (1983) Maternal nutritional status and adolescent pregnancy outcome. *American Journal of Clinical Nutrition* **38**: 739–46

Gardosi J, Chang A, Kalyan B, Sahota D, Symonds EM (1992) Customised antenatal growth charts. *Lancet* **339**: 283–87

Gardosi J, Clausson B, Francis A (2009) The value of customised centiles in assessing perinatal mortality risk associated with parity and maternal size. *British Journal of Obstetrics and Gynaecology* **116**: 1356–63

Gardosi J, Kady SM, McGeown P, Francis A, Tonks A (2005) Classification of stillbirth by relevant condition at death (ReCoDe): Population based cohort study. *British Medical Journal* **331**(7525): 1113–7

Gilbert WM, Nesbitt TS, Danielsen B (1999) Childbearing beyond age 40: Pregnancy outcome in 24,032 cases. *Obstetrics and Gynecology* **93**(1): 9–14

Gutierrez Y, King JC (1993) Nutrition during teenage pregnancy. *Pediatric Annals* **22**: 99–108

Han SN, Van Calsteren K, Heyns L, Mhallem Gziri M, Amant F (2010) Breast cancer during pregnancy: a literature review. *Minerva Ginecol* **62**(6): 585–97

Hasegawa J, Matsuoka R, Ichizuka K et al (2009) Predisposing factors for massive hemorrhage during cesarean section in patients with placenta previa. *Ultrasound Obstetrics and Gynecology* **34**(1): 80–4

Hayward CE, Greenwood SL, Sibley CP, Baker PN, Challis JRG, Jones RL (2011a) Effect of maternal age and growth on placental nutrient transport: Potential mechanisms for teenagers' predisposition to small-for-gestational-age birth? *American Journal of Physiology Endocrinolology and Metabolism* [Epub ahead of print]

Hayward CE, Greenwood SL, Sibley CP, Baker PN, Jones RL (2011b) Effect of young maternal age and skeletal growth on placental growth and development. *Placenta* **32**: 990–98

Hediger ML, Scholl TO, Belsky DH, Ances IG, Salmon RW (1989) Patterns of weight gain in adolescent pregnancy: Effects on birth weight and preterm delivery. *Obstetrics and Gynecology* **74**: 6–12

Hediger ML, Scholl TO, Schall JI, Krueger PM (1997) Young maternal age and preterm labor. *Annals of Epidemiology* **7**: 400–6

Heffner LJ, Elkin E, Fretts RC (2003) Impact of labor induction, gestational age, and maternal age on cesarean delivery rates. *Obstetrics and Gynecology* **102**(2): 287–93

Henne MB, Zhang M, Paroski S, Kelshikar B, Westphal LM (2007) Comparison of obstetric outcomes in recipients of donor oocytes vs. women of advanced maternal age with autologous oocytes. *Journal of Reproductive Medicine* **52**(7): 585–90

Hijaz A, Sadeghi Z, Byrne L, Hou JC, Daneshgari F (2012) Advanced maternal age as a risk factor for stress urinary incontinence: A review of the literature. I*nternational Urogynecology Journal* **23**(4): 395–401

Hornemann A, Kamischke A, Luedders DW, Beyer DA, Diedrich K, Bohlmann MK (2010) Advanced age is a risk factor for higher grade perineal lacerations during delivery in nulliparous women. *Archives of Gynecology and Obstetrics* **281**(1): 59–64

Huang L, Sauve R, Birkett N, Fergusson D, van Walraven C (2008) Maternal age and risk of stillbirth: A systematic review. *Canadian Medical Association Journal* **178**(2): 165–72

Igwegbe AO, Udigwe GO (2001) Teenage pregnancy: Still an obstetric risk. *Journal of Obstetrics and Gynaecology* **21**: 478–81

Institute of Medicine (2009) *Weight gain during pregnancy: Reexamining the guidelines*. The National Academies Press, Washington DC

Ip M, Peyman E, Lohsoonthorn V, Williams MA (2010) A case-control study of preterm delivery risk factors according to clinical subtypes and severity. *Journal of Obstetric and Gynaecology Research* **36**(1): 34–44

Jacobsson B, Ladfors L, Milsom I (2004) Advanced maternal age and adverse perinatal outcome. *Obstetrics and Gynecology* **104**(4): 727–33

Jolly MC, Sebire N, Harris J, Robinson S, Regan L (2000a) Obstetric risks of pregnancy in women less than 18 years old. *Obstetrics and Gynecology* **96**: 962–6

Jolly M, Sebire N, Harris J, Robinson S, Regan L (2000b) The risks associated with pregnancy in women aged 35 years or older. *Human Reproduction* **15**(11): 2433–7

Jones RL et al (2010) Relationship between maternal growth, infant birthweight and nutrient partitioning in teenage pregnancies. *British Journal of Obstetrics and Gynaecology* **117**: 200–11

Khashan AS, Baker PN, Kenny LC (2010) Preterm birth and reduced birthweight in first and second teenage pregnancies: A register-based cohort study. *BMC Pregnancy Childbirth* **10**: 1–8

Kim C, Newton KM, Knopp RH (2002) Gestational diabetes and the incidence of type 2 diabetes: A systematic review. *Diabetes Care* **25**(10): 1862–8

Knight MSP, Fitzpatrick K, Misztela D, Acosta C, Kurinczuk JJ (2011) *United Kingdom Obstetric Surveillance System (UKOSS) Annual Report 2011.* National Perinatal Epidemiology Unit, Oxford

Knopp R (1997) Hormone-mediated changes in nutrient metabolism in pregnancy: A physiological basis for normal fetal development. *Annals of the New York Academy of Science* **817**: 251–71

Lambers D, Clark K (1996) The maternal and fetal physiologic effects of nicotine. *Seminars in Perinatology* **20**: 115–26

Lenders CM, McElrath TF, Scholl TO (2000) Nutrition in adolescent pregnancy. *Current Opinions in Pediatrics* **12**: 291–6

Liu K, Case A (2011) Advanced reproductive age and fertility. *Journal of Obstetrics and Gynaecology Canada* **33**(11): 1165–75

Loke AY, Poon CF (2011) The health concerns and behaviours of primigravida: Comparing advanced age pregnant women with their younger counterparts. *Journal of Clinical Nursing* **20**(7–8): 1141–50

MacKay DF, Smith GC, Dobbie R, Pell JP (2010) Gestational age at delivery and special educational need: Retrospective cohort study of 407,503 schoolchildren. *PLoS Medicine* **7**(6): e1000289

Mackie FL, Taylor CE, Greenwood SL, Jones RL (2011) Impact of poor nutritional status on placental development and function in teenage pregnancy. *Archives of Diseases in Childhood - Fetal Neonatalal Education* **96**: Fa54

Mahomed K, Bhutta Z, Middleton P (2007) Zinc supplementation for improving pregnancy and infant outcome. *Cochrane Database of Systematic Reviews* CD000230

Mahony R, Enright F, O'Herlihy C, Foley ME (2009) Cerebral palsy following neonatal hypoxic seizures in singleton term infants: The influence of parity. *Irish Medical Journal* **102**(8): 246–9

Makrides M, Crowther C (2001) Magnesium supplementation in pregnancy. *Cochrane Database of Systematic Reviews* CD000937

Malouf AJ, Norton CS, Engel AF, Nicholls RJ, Kamm MA (2000) Long-term results of overlapping anterior anal-sphincter repair for obstetric trauma. *Lancet* **355**(9200): 260–5

Maman E, Lunenfeld E, Levy A, Vardi H, Potashnik G (1998) Obstetric outcome of singleton pregnancies conceived by in vitro fertilization and ovulation induction compared with those conceived spontaneously. *Fertility and Sterility* 70(2): 240–5

Maxwell GL (1993) Preterm premature rupture of membranes. *Obstetrics and Gynecology Surveys* **48**(8): 576–83

McMahon CA, Boivin J, Gibson FL, Fisher JR, Hammarberg K, Wynter K, Saunders DM (2011) Older first-time mothers and early postpartum depression: A prospective cohort study of women conceiving spontaneously or with assisted reproductive technologies. *Fertility and Sterility* **96**(5): 1218–24

McVeigh JKJJ (2007) *Perinatal risks associated with IVF. Scientific Advisory Committee Opinion Paper 8.* RCOG Press, London

Metzger BE, Lowe LP, Dyer AR et al (2008). Hyperglycemia and adverse pregnancy outcomes. *New England Journal of Medicine* **358**(19): 1991–2002

Mills JL, Scott JM, Kirke PN et al (1996) Homocysteine and neural tube defects. *Journal of Nutrition* **126**: 756S–60S

Montan S (2007) Increased risk in the elderly parturient. *Current Opinion in Obstetrics and Gynecology* **19**(2): 110–2

Moran VH (2007) A systematic review of dietary assessments of pregnant adolescents in industrialised countries. *British Journal of Nutrition* **97**: 411–25

Morris JK, Wald NJ, Mutton DE, Alberman E (2003) Comparison of models of maternal age-specific risk for Down syndrome live births. *Prenatal Diagnosis* **23**(3): 252–8

National Collaborating Centre for Mental Health (2007) *Antenatal and postnatal mental health.* In: Society BP (ed.) Alden Press, London

National Collaborating Centre for Women's and Children's Health (2008a) *Diabetes in pregnancy: Management of diabetes and its complications from preconception to the postnatal period.* National Institute for Clinical Excellence, London

National Collaborating Centre for Women's and Children's Health (2008b) *Induction of labour.* National Institute for Clinical Excellence, London

National Collaborating Centre for Women's and Children's Health (2011) *Hypertension in pregnancy: The management of hypertensive disorders during pregnancy.* RCOG Press, London

National Collaborating Centre for Women's and Children's Health (2004) *Fertility: Assessment and treatment for people with fertility problems.* RCOG Press, London

National Collaborating Centre for Women's and Children's Health (2008) *Antenatal care: Routine care for the health of pregnant woman.* Royal College of Obstetricians and Gynaecologists Press, London

National Collaborating Centre for Women's and Children's Health (2010) *Pregnancy and complex social factors: A model for service provision for pregnant women with complex social factors.* Royal College of Obstetrics and Gynaecologists, London

Nielsen JN, Gittelsohn J, Anliker J, O'Brien K (2006) Interventions to improve diet and weight gain among pregnant adolescents and recommendations for future research. *Journal of the American Dietetic Association* **106**: 1825–40

Nybo AA, Wohlfahrt J, Christens P, Olsen J, Melbye M (2000) Is maternal age an independent risk factor for fetal loss? *Western Journal of Medicine* **173**(5): 331

Pasquier JC, Picaud JC, Rabilloud M, et al (2009) Neonatal outcomes after elective delivery management of preterm premature rupture of the membranes before 34 weeks' gestation (DOMINOS study). *European Journal of Obstetrics and Gynecology Reproductive Biology* **143**(1): 18–23

Pentheroudakis G, Pavlidis N (2006) Cancer and pregnancy: Poena magna, not anymore. *European Journal of Cancer* **42**(2): 126–40

Pereg D, Koren G, Lishner M (2008) Cancer in pregnancy: Gaps, challenges and solutions. *Cancer Treatment Reviews* **34**(4): 302–12

Porreco RP, Harden L, Gambotto M, Shapiro H (2005) Expectation of pregnancy outcome among mature women. *American Journal of Obstetrics and Gynecology* **192**(1): 38–41

Raymond EG, Cnattingius S, Kiely JL (1994) Effects of maternal age, parity, and smoking on the risk of stillbirth. *British Journal of Obstetrics and Gynaecology* **101**(4): 301–6

Reddy UM, Ko, CW, Willinger M (2006) Maternal age and the risk of stillbirth throughout pregnancy in the United States. *American Journal of Obstetrics and Gynecology* **195**(3): 764–70

Reefhuis J, Honein MA (2004) Maternal age and non-chromosomal birth defects, Atlanta1968–2000: Teenager or thirty-something, who is at risk? *Birth Defects Research. Part A, Clinical and Molecular Teratology* **70**(9): 572–9

Rioux FM, LeBlanc CP (2007) Iron supplementation during pregnancy: What are the risks and benefits of current practices? *Applied Physiology and Nutritional Metabolism* **32**: 282–8

Roos N, Sahlin L, Ekman-Ordeberg G, Kieler H, Stephansson O (2010) Maternal risk factors for postterm pregnancy and cesarean delivery following labor induction. *Acta Obstetrica and Gynecologica Scandinavica* **89**(8): 1003–10

Rumbold A, Crowther C (2005a) Vitamin C supplementation in pregnancy. *Cochrane Database of Systematics Reviews* CD004072

Rumbold A, Crowther C (2005b) Vitamin E supplementation in pregnancy. *Cochrane Database of Systematic Reviews* CD004069

Saigal S, Doyle LW (2008) An overview of mortality and sequelae of preterm birth from infancy to adulthood. *Lancet* **371**(9608): 261–9

Salihu HM, Shumpert MN, Slay M, Kirby RS, Alexander GR (2003) Childbearing beyond maternal age 50 and fetal outcomes in the United States. *Obstetrics and Gynecology* **102**(5 Pt 1): 1006–14

Satin AJ, Leveno KJ, Sherman ML, Reedy NJ, Lowe TW, McIntire DD (1994) Maternal youth and pregnancy outcomes: Middle school versus high school age groups compared with women beyond the teen years. *American Journal of Obstetrics and Gynecology* **171**: 184–7

Schoen C, Rosen T (2009) Maternal and perinatal risks for women over 44 – a review. *Maturitas* **64**(2): 109–13

Scholl TO, Hediger ML, Ances IG (1990) Maternal growth during pregnancy and decreased infant birth weight. *American Journal of Clinical Nutrition* **51**: 790–3

Scholl TO, Hediger ML, Schall JI, Khoo CS, Fischer RL (1994) Maternal growth during pregnancy and the competition for nutrients. *American Journal of Clinical Nutrition* **60**: 183–8

Scholl TO, Hediger ML, Schall JI, Khoo CS, Fischer RL (1996) Dietary and serum folate: Their influence on the outcome of pregnancy. *American Journal of Clinical Nutrition* 63: 520–5

Sheiner E, Shoham-Vardi I, Hallak M, et al (2003) Placental abruption in term pregnancies: Clinical significance and obstetric risk factors. *Journal of Maternal and Fetal Neonatal Medicine* **13**(1): 45–9

Shrim A, Levin I, Mallozzi A, et al (2010) Does very advanced maternal age, with or without egg donation, really increase obstetric risk in a large tertiary center? *Journal of Perinatal Medicine* **38**(6): 645–50

Sibai BM (2002) Chronic hypertension in pregnancy. *Obstetrics and Gynecology* **100**(2): 369–77

Smith GC, Cordeaux Y, White IR, et al (2008) The effect of delaying childbirth on primary cesarean section rates. *PLoS Medicine* **5**(7): e144

Smith GCS, Pell JP (2001) Teenage pregnancy and risk of adverse perinatal outcomes associated with first and second births: Population based retrospective cohort study. *British Medical Journal* **323**: 476–9

Stang J, Story MT, Harnack L, Neumark-Sztainer D (2000) Relationships between vitamin and mineral supplement use, dietary intake, and dietary adequacy among adolescents. *Journal of the American Dietetic Association* **100**: 905–10

Stein Z, Susser M (2000) The risks of having children in later life. Social advantage may make up for biological disadvantage. *British Medical Journal* **320**(7251): 1681–2

Tallo CP, Vohr B, Oh W, Rubin LP, Seifer DB, Haning RVJr. (1995) Maternal and neonatal morbidity associated with in vitro fertilization. *Journal of Pediatrics* **127**(5): 794–800

Tan SL, Doyle P, Campbell S, et al (1992). Obstetric outcome of in vitro fertilization pregnancies compared with normally conceived pregnancies. *American Journal of Obstetrics and Gynecology* **167**(3): 778–84

Thaver D, Saeed M, Bhutta Z (2006) Pyridoxine (vitamin B6) suppplementation in pregnancy. *Cochrane Database of Systematic Reviews* CD000179

Treacy A, Robson, M, O'Herlihy C (2006) Dystocia increases with advancing maternal age. *American Journal of Obstetrics and Gynecology* **195**(3): 760–3

Tsur A, Sergienko R, Wiznitzer A, Zlotnik A, Sheiner E (2011) Critical analysis of risk factors for shoulder dystocia. *Archives of Gynecology and Obstetrics* **285**(5): 1225–9

Valachis A, Tsali L, Pesce LL, Polyzos NP, Dimitriadis C, Tsalis K, Mauri D (2010) Safety of pregnancy after primary breast carcinoma in young women: A meta-analysis to overcome bias of healthy mother effect studies. *Obstetrics and Gynecology Surveys* **65**(12): 786–93

Valdimarsdottir U, Hultman CM, Harlow B, Cnattingius S, Sparen P (2009) Psychotic illness in first-time mothers with no previous psychiatric hospitalizations: A population-based study. *PLoS Medicine* **6**(2): e13

Viau PA, Padula CA, Eddy B (2002) An exploration of health concerns and health-promotion behaviors in pregnant women over age 35. *MCN American Journal of Maternal Child Nursing* **27**(6): 328–34

Vigil-De Gracia P, Montufar-Rueda C, Smith A (2004) Pregnancy and severe chronic hypertension: Maternal outcome. *Hypertension in Pregnancy* **23**(3): 285–93

Wahl R (1999) Nutrition in adolescence. *Pediatric Annals* **28**: 107–11

Wang JX, Clark AM, Kirby CA, et al (1994) The obstetric outcome of singleton pregnancies following in-vitro fertilization/gamete intra-fallopian transfer. *Human Reproduction* **9**(1): 141–6

Wild J, Sutcliffe M, Schorah CJ, Levene MI (1997) Prevention of neural-tube defects. *Lancet* **350**: 30–1

World Health Organization (1992) *The prevalence of anaemia in women: A tabulation of available information.* World Health Organization, Geneva

Wu S, Kocherginsky M, Hibbard JU (2005) Abnormal placentation: Twenty-year analysis. *American Journal of Obstetrics and Gynecology* **192**(5): 1458–61

Yang J, Savitz DA, Dole N, Hartmann KE, Herring AH, Olshan AF, Thorp JM Jr. (2005) Predictors of vaginal bleeding during the first two trimesters of pregnancy. *Paediatric and Perinatal Epidemiology* **19**(4): 276–83

Yogev Y, Melamed N, Bardin R, Tenenbaum-Gavish K, Ben-Shitrit G, Ben-Haroush A (2010) Pregnancy outcome at extremely advanced maternal age. *American Journal of Obstetrics and Gynecology* **203**(6): 558 e1–7

Zhu BP, Rolfs RT, Nangle BE, Horan J (1999) Effect of the interval between pregnancies on perinatal outcomes. *New England Journal of Medicine* **349**: 589–94

Zwart JJ, Richters JM, Ory F, de Vries JI, Bloemenkamp KW, van Roosmalen J (2009) Uterine rupture in The Netherlands: A nationwide population-based cohort study. *British Journal of Obstetrics and Gynaecology* **116**(8): 1069–78; discussion 1078–80

Chapter 4

Supporting younger and older women during pregnancy and birth

Introduction

This chapter focuses on support during pregnancy and birth for teenagers and women of advanced maternal age. Improving attendance at antenatal appointments is crucial to the provision of effective care for pregnant teenagers. Using the example of a well-established clinic for teenagers, the best ways to meet the specific needs of this age group are discussed and recommendations made for best practice. In caring for older women, midwives need to consider particular issues related to advancing maternal age, including the increased incidence of poor outcomes. Section 2 considers specific issues related to the care of older women, including prevention and detection of complications and the need for specialist care pathways. Current guidance on care for women of advanced maternal age will also be discussed.

Section 1
Care of the pregnant teenager

Sue Thompson and Lorna Wood

I am good, but not an angel.
I do sin, but I'm not the devil.
I am just a small girl in a big world trying to find someone to love.

Marilyn Monroe

Introduction

The responsibility of the midwife involved in providing antenatal care for pregnant teenagers is diverse. The midwife has to be able to make routine assessments in terms of monitoring pregnancy, antenatal education and safe parenting. However, midwives also need an awareness of the diversity of teenage lifestyles and they need expertise in other areas, especially around safeguarding and consent. This will enable them to highlight any areas of concern and allow for monitoring and re-visiting of social situations that may impact on pregnancy and parenting. Any concerns can be discussed with the safeguarding lead within the NHS trust and a social services referral can be made if necessary.

Antenatal care should maximise positive clinical outcomes as well as provide support and reassurance through monitoring (Department of Health, 2004). The National Institute for Health and Clinical Excellence (NICE) recommends 10 antenatal appointments for nulliparous and seven for parous women (NICE, 2008). However, flexibility should be exercised when looking after younger women as their social, financial and family circumstances often change and their physical and psychological needs are difficult to define at booking. The key elements of continuity of midwifery care are particularly relevant for pregnant teenagers, including having the time to talk, and engaging in and building relationships with women, their partners and other family members to understand and help meet their needs throughout pregnancy and afterwards (Department of Health, 2007).

The latest NICE guideline for women with complex social needs (NICE, 2010a) recognises that pregnant teenagers are a special group of young women requiring specialist midwifery care.

Complexities of supporting teenagers in pregnancy

The Young Women's Clinic was set up in Liverpool over 15 years ago by midwife Lorna Wood, who recognised that the existing obstetric service was not meeting the needs of pregnant teenagers. At that time, teenagers were seen in general antenatal clinics. Lorna worked with a female consultant obstetrician, who was also interested in teenage pregnancy and who was keen to support the plan for the midwifery-led clinic. In 1994, all young women who were under 18 years of age were identified from antenatal booking letters and were given appointments to attend the Young Women's Clinic.

The Young Women's Clinic has since been run by Sue Thompson, Teenage Pregnancy Midwife. The following section uses this clinic as a basis to discuss the antenatal care of young parents.

Background

The clinic was planned in 1992 in response to several triggers affecting antenatal services in Liverpool at that time: the amalgamation of two maternity hospitals;

the reorganisation of parent education and community services; and anecdotal evidence from midwives that pregnant teenagers tended to book late, default from the antenatal clinic and were less likely to attend parent education classes. This led to a review of the literature which suggested that there were different risks for younger and older teenagers, supporting the view that a service should be set up specifically for younger pregnant teenagers (Russell, 1988; Hedger et al, 1989; Konje et al, 1992). The review included a search of local and national policies and resulted in the recognition that there was very little guidance at that time for midwifery care for this group of pregnant women. Nevertheless, there was an acknowledgment that teenage pregnancy and a reduction in teenage conceptions should be a Department of Health target (Department of Health, 1992).

Within the literature, risks of teenage pregnancy were identified predominantly as medical risks, such as anaemia, preterm labour, intrauterine growth restriction and infant mortality (Konje et al, 1992; Fraser et al, 1995; Miller et al, 1996). However, there was an increasing recognition of the association between socioeconomic deprivation as both a cause and a consequence of teenage parenthood (Simms and Smith, 1986; Smith, 1993; Keirnan, 1995). The review ultimately secured funding for a specialist midwife for pregnant teenagers in Liverpool.

Referrals to the clinic were established by informing all general practitioners and midwives within the Liverpool city boundary of the service. The clinic was held on a different day from the routine antenatal clinics, to acknowledge the possible barriers that could be created by perceptions of disapproval from older mothers-to-be and their families, and with the aim that teenagers might feel more relaxed by attending with their peers. Teenagers in Liverpool followed the national trend of booking late and not attending for routine antenatal care (Bristol Booking Survey, 1983; Simms and Smith, 1984). Before the specialist clinic, teenagers were also less likely to attend parent education classes and often presented in labour with very little preparation or knowledge about the process of birth, breastfeeding or parenting. As a result, young women were often unprepared for the reality of giving birth and breastfeeding (Dewan et al, 2002).

Young partners were also unsure of what their role was during pregnancy and labour and there was often tension between partners and parents, making pregnancy and birth stressful for all involved. The new service for young pregnant women aimed to address this within the care pathway planned at the booking visit. This crucial early access and continuity of care helped to build a trusting relationship between the young woman, her partner, parents and the Teenage Pregnancy Midwife.

The complexities of teenage pregnancy

Issues pertinent to teenage parents are complicated and revolve around age, emotional maturity, relationships with parents and partners, social and safeguarding problems, and educational needs. The relationships between these factors and pregnancy are complex and there is mounting evidence that dislike of school, in particular, is associated with social disadvantage and unintended pregnancy, and this may be exacerbated by complicated family problems and social issues (Kiernan, 1995; Bonell et al, 2005; Wiggins et al, 2005).

Young women attending the clinic are encouraged to stay in education, either through home tuition or college courses. Within the clinic, the needs of younger teenagers (14 to 17-year-olds) have been identified as different in many aspects to those of older teenagers (18 and 19-year-olds), particularly in terms of emotional maturity, financial independence and shortened educational experience (Edwards, 2000). Young parents often have unstable and volatile relationships with their partners, which may be a significant cause of stress during pregnancy (Department for Children, Schools and Families, 2008).

Emotional uncertainty can have negative physical and psychological impacts on pregnancy; women often report being unable to relax, and having increasing feelings of isolation. Women living in families with high unemployment are also likely to suffer increased poverty and social exclusion, which can increase the risk of developing depression (Department of Health, 2007). Moreover, teenage mothers are three times more likely than older mothers to develop postnatal depression, and when teenage mothers reach 30 years of age they are 22% more likely to be living in poverty than mothers giving birth aged 24 or over. They are also less likely to be living with a partner or to be employed (Ermisch and Pevalin, 2003).

Access to services

Reasons for poor attendance at antenatal clinic, accessing services later in pregnancy and failure to attend parent education classes are well documented (Department of Health, 2004; Teenage Pregnancy Unit, 2004; NICE 2010a). Pregnant teenagers fail to access maternity services for a number of reasons; they may not realise that they are pregnant and there may be psychological barriers to coming to terms with pregnancy. Many teenagers have fears about the reaction of the family, and other social issues, in terms of housing, take priority, and financial worries may make transportation to clinics difficult (Department of Health, 2004; Teenage Pregnancy Unit, 2004; NICE 2010a). Pregnant teenagers and young fathers often feel self-conscious using services where older service users are present. They are particularly sensitive to the possibility of encountering criticism, especially when using maternity services.

Acknowledging these barriers, the philosophy of the Young Women's Clinic is based on a holistic, non-judgemental care package. This can be achieved as the midwives involved in the clinic are genuinely interested in caring for teenagers. This may seem an obvious assumption to make, but not all midwives have an interest in or the aptitude for providing care for this group of women, and this is fundamental in terms of the trust needed to make the relationship work. The clinic is held in the afternoon, a deliberate arrangement to fit in with the teenage lifestyle of getting up late and poor attendance at morning appointments. There is also a welcoming environment from all staff, with positive images of young mothers and fathers displayed.

Continuity of care

The Young Women's Clinic offers continuity of care for the young woman, her partner and her family, by a named midwife with expertise in teenage pregnancy, sexual health, contraception and teenage parenting. With this approach, the clinic has a very low non-attendance rate.

This approach is supported by several studies that have identified a positive association between healthy pregnancy outcomes and support given in pregnancy (Clemmens, 2001; Goyder et al, 2003; Swann et al, 2003; Furey, 2004). In order to enhance that support, all teenagers attending the clinic have access to the teenage pregnancy midwife via a mobile (work) telephone. All young women, their partners and parents have access to the midwife's phone number and can contact her during working hours (Department for Children, Schools and Families, 2008). The midwife will often suggest texting her (to reduce costs) and she will ring back, allowing all teenagers equal access to midwifery support, irrespective of income. Young women and partners are offered the option of individual, 'one-to-one' parent education sessions if they wish, which avoids embarrassing situations. For example, the young person may not understand what is being discussed but feels unable to speak out (in a group) and is left feeling frustrated and demoralised. This one-to-one approach encourages clarity and open communication.

Social history

The Young Women's Clinic has always collected additional social history information, which is documented in the hospital casenotes at the booking visit. This extra information enables the midwife to signpost teenagers to appropriate support. The data gathered include information about use of contraception; whether the pregnancy was planned or unplanned; and, depending on age, whether or not the school is aware, if home tuition is needed, and plans for future education. Domestic arrangements are recorded including current address, who the young woman lives with, where she is planning to live after the birth, who accompanied her to the booking visit and whether or not her parents are aware of the pregnancy. Details about the partner's involvement, including his name, age and whether he has any other children are also sought. A record of current or past social work involvement is made, including whether the young woman or her partner are, or have ever been, 'looked after children'. The history provides crucial information which contributes to the assessment of how much support each teenager will need throughout pregnancy and after the birth of the baby.

This information is updated regularly as the pregnancy progresses and provides an ongoing audit for the service. Partner information, particularly age of partner and whether or not he has fathered other children can often be a trigger for safeguarding concerns. Whilst asking questions within the social history, emotional and social vulnerability can be gauged by the answers given. Examples of the family support questions asked often follow a line of enquiry such as the relationship with the mother, who else lives at home, where and with whom are they planning to stay after the birth and whether they will be sharing a bedroom.

Social information is pertinent to assessing what extra support is needed, as the children of teenage mothers have a 63% increased risk of being born into poverty compared to babies born to mothers in their 20s (Mayhew and Bradshaw, 2005), and have higher mortality rates under eight years old (Corbin, 2004). Children born to the most vulnerable teenagers are at an increased risk (nearly one in three) of becoming teenage mothers themselves (Wellings et al, 2001).

Pregnancy complications such as fetal growth restriction are linked to diet and social behaviour, particularly smoking (Dewan et al, 2003). Teenage mothers are three times more likely to smoke throughout pregnancy than older mothers (Bolling et al, 2007) and 50% less likely to breastfeed, both of which have negative health consequences for the child (Department of Health, 2007).

Diet

Antenatal care should include a dietary review, since good maternal nutrition before and during pregnancy is key for optimum pregnancy outcome. Many pregnant teenagers have an inadequate dietary intake of nutrients, and unhealthy, often erratic, eating patterns (Burchet and Seeley, 2003). Most pregnant teenagers under 18 years of age are not eligible for means tested benefits until the last 11 weeks of pregnancy. When teenagers no longer live with their parents, the risks of poor diet are increased because of limited cooking facilities, lack of knowledge and experience, and financial constraints (Dallison and Lobstein, 1995, Burchet and Seeley 2003).

Pregnant teenagers up to the age of 18 years are currently eligible for UK Government Healthy Start vouchers which enable the purchase of milk, fresh or frozen fruit and vegetables and infant formula milk. The Healthy Start booklet is discussed and given at the first visit to the Young Women's Clinic to enable the teenager to start claiming her vouchers. Importantly, a new claim must be made once the baby is born, and a sticker is included in the postnatal notes to remind young parents to re-claim for this vital support. The midwives offer advice about healthy diet during pregnancy as part of the routine antenatal care and within the parenting classes (Department of Health, 2008).

Exercise

NICE Guidelines (2008) advise that moderate exercise in pregnancy can be undertaken, whilst being aware of potential dangers of high impact contact sports or scuba diving, the latter being associated with fetal birth defects and disease. Beginning and continuing a moderate course of exercise during pregnancy is not associated with adverse outcomes, and pelvic floor exercises should be encouraged. Information and advice relevant to exercise, particularly pelvic floor exercise, is discussed as part of the routine antenatal information at booking.

Parent education

As well as reduced engagement with clinical care, teenage mothers and young fathers are also much less likely than older parents to attend for parent education. Teenagers often state that they feel uncomfortable in classes dominated by older women and women with husbands or partners, and much prefer classes targeted at their own age group (Department for Children, Schools and Families, 2008). A rolling programme of classes is offered, involving four sessions covering:

- Onset of labour and pain relief (including how to cope at home in early labour).
- Stages of labour and coping mechanisms in hospital and for home birth.
- A tour of the hospital delivery suite, midwifery led-unit, birthing pool and postnatal wards.
- Bathing baby, routine vaccinations and going home with baby.

These classes are offered at the same time as antenatal care, as teenagers are less likely to come back to a separate session. The sessions last for one hour at lunch time. All teenagers can opt to attend the class or have one-to-one sessions if they are uncomfortable in a group situation.

Babies need fathers

A good relationship between a young father and his teenage partner during pregnancy is strongly correlated with his involvement with his child in the early years (bootcampfornewdads.org). A positive relationship between mother and father is also a protective factor for postnatal depression, and a father's attitudes to the mother breastfeeding and to giving up smoking have been found to have a very strong influence on the mother (Department for Children, Schools and Families, 2008). Indeed, it is often because the young father wants his baby to have the very best start in life that he will encourage his partner to breastfeed and be willing to support her in every way he can to facilitate this. Conversely, the young father may not want to 'share' his partner with the demands of a newborn and if he does not want her to breastfeed, it is unlikely she will do so (Department for Children, Schools and Families, 2008).

Specific efforts are made to reach out to young men by involving them in antenatal care and by giving them the sense that they are respected and valued in their role, so that they do not disengage from the pregnancy or parenting. The clinic encourages young men to feel 'included' from the first visit by warmly acknowledging their importance in the pregnancy and birth, by making eye contact and by asking their opinion and valuing what they say in response.

All teenage fathers are invited to a unique workshop 'Hit the ground crawling' (bootcampfornewdads.org). This is a specific three-hour workshop for young 'dads to be' in which they learn what to expect from labour and birth. Other topics covered include why babies cry, and how to care for a crying baby and a stressed mother. Practical advice on changing a baby's nappy and bathing is included and 10 top tips for dads include awareness of common symptoms of postnatal depression. Information is also given on resuming sex and contraception. Most importantly this workshop reinforces how vitally important fathers can be in their baby's life.

Breastfeeding

Breastfeeding has a strong protective effect on the health of both baby and mother. Babies who are not breastfed are at increased risk of gastrointestinal, middle ear and urine infections, childhood diabetes and obesity (Dyson et al, 2006). Mothers who do not breastfeed are at increased risk of ovarian and pre-menopausal breast cancer (Bolling et al, 2007). Moreover, teenagers are less likely to breastfeed than older women and those who do initiate breastfeeding are likely to end it sooner. One study found that only 34% of teenagers were still breastfeeding one week after the birth and only 7% at six months; this was five times lower than the rate for women aged 35 and over (Bolling et al, 2007).

In 2001 the Young Women's Clinic secured funding from the Department of Health (Department of Health, 2001) for one year to identify and support all teenagers who planned to breastfeed their babies. The 'Breastfeeding Guardian for Teenagers' project offered all teenagers the intervention of one-to-one breastfeeding support from a midwife (guardian). This service was additional to the midwifery care from the Young Women's Clinic. The guardian offered support throughout the antenatal, intrapartum and postnatal period whilst in hospital. On discharge, all teenagers were encouraged to keep a diary (best and worst experiences of feeding that day and week) and to contact the guardian by text or phone when they felt in need of support to continue breastfeeding. The guardian also contacted them either on a daily or weekly basis, depending on need, to encourage and support.

The guardian was able to provide a unique, individual service to the young women and their babies that improved initiation and continuation of breastfeeding. For example, one of the youngest teenagers, aged 15, breastfed her baby until he was 14 months old. There was also a snowball effect in that other issues were uncovered during this time, such as advice on fear of resuming sexual contact after birth, contraception, changing body image, housing, relationships and how to trust others caring for the baby (Lavender et al, 2005).

Conclusion

> *Immature love says:'I love you because I need you'. Mature love says:'I need you because I love you.'*
>
> (Erich Fromm)

Pregnant teenagers and young fathers often feel self-conscious and afraid when using adult services. They may have experienced disapproving comments and are often very sensitive to the possibility of encountering criticism when using maternity services. Creating a welcoming environment and specialist midwifery services is vitally important to reassure young people that maternity services are 'for them'.

The following case studies are based on true teenage pregnancy stories with the use of pseudonyms.

Case study 4.1

Gemma was 15 years old, in year 10 at school, and was accompanied to the Young Women's Antenatal Clinic by her parents. She had come to 'book in' because she'd just discovered that she was 13 weeks pregnant. She had initially intended to have a termination of pregnancy and had attended for the counselling process prior to going through with the procedure, but changed her mind at the last moment.

Gemma was an only child and her parents both worked full time. They were distraught at their daughter's decision to continue with the pregnancy and all three were upset and in tears during the initial consultation. Her father was angry and he and his wife felt that their daughter was too young to cope with a baby,. She hadn't finished her education and they wanted her to have the pregnancy terminated. Neither he nor his wife could afford to give up work to look after a baby and they did not want to do this anyway.

Questions and discussion points

- Parental concerns are an important aspect of the decision making process. What influences pregnant teenagers to be able to make informed decisions about continuing with the pregnancy or opting for termination?
- Why do parents need to feel that their opinions are important?
- How could the midwife, as an advocate for teenagers, facilitate this dialogue so that they all have a chance to express their fears, concerns and opinions?

- In this case study, the partner was not part of the discussion. How could the midwife have provided an opportunity to identify and support his needs and fears?

Action taken by the midwife

The midwife asked the parents to wait outside for a few moments and spoke to Gemma privately and asked her what she really wanted to do about the pregnancy. Importantly, did she want to continue and was she under any threat or being pressured by anyone else in making this decision? She was adamant that it was her own choice and she wanted to keep her baby. Her boyfriend was also 15 years old and he had left the decision up to her.

When her parents returned to the room, the midwife explained the situation and the girl's father became angry and upset again saying, 'So you are telling me that this 15-year-old girl can make that decision; she has no means of looking after herself, never mind a baby, but she has the final say on something as profound as this?'

All the midwife could do was respond by reiterating that this was Gemma's decision.

The midwife can only offer advice and support. Gemma's father was relieved when the midwife explained that, because of her age, Gemma would be fully supported to return to education and the baby would be given a free place at a nursery (or child-minder) of their own choosing. This package of support, called Care to Learn, is funded by the Government and would be available until Gemma reaches the age of 20.

This information helped Gemma's parents to calm down enough for a productive and meaningful conversation to take place. Gemma was relieved to hear about the scheme as she wanted to continue with her education and had not wanted to be a 'burden' to her parents.

Case study 4.2

Sophie, aged 16, attended the clinic with her partner James, aged 17. She was 28 weeks pregnant and her 20 week scan had confirmed that all was well with the pregnancy. Sophie looked pale and was wrapped in a few layers of clothing, including a woolly hat. Her body mass index (BMI) was 18.5 at booking. During the antenatal appointment, the midwife asked her how she was feeling, if the baby had been moving every day, as well as the usual questions. Sophie reassured the midwife that all was well and the baby moved a lot every day and her appetite was normal. Nevertheless, the midwife decided to pursue this further and asked her, 'What have you had to eat today?' (It was 4.00 p.m.) 'Oh nothing yet' was the reply. The midwife asked her if she'd had anything to drink and she admitted she'd had a bottle of energy drink and a can of Pepsi.

Questions and discussion points

- What causes barriers to be created during a midwifery consultation with a pregnant teenager?
- How can these barriers be avoided or overcome?
- What aspects of communication are vital when caring for pregnant teenagers and their partners?
- How can the midwife ensure that communication is successful?

Action taken by the midwife

The midwife asked Sophie if she planned to eat later (at her mother's house perhaps) and she shrugged her shoulders and said 'probably'. Her partner had remained sitting in the chair, quietly staring at the floor. It was obvious that all was not well with this couple and so the midwife asked more direct questions. It appeared that James' mother had presumed he would be moving in with Sophie at her mother's house (as he spent a lot of time there already). His bedroom was now being used for another family member, so when James wanted to stay at his home, his 'bed' was now on the settee in the living room. James felt that his family were not really interested in him or in supporting the young couple and their baby.

Sophie currently shared her bedroom with her younger sister and felt guilty that her sister would have no room to sleep in once the baby arrived. Sophie felt her mother was angry with her for creating this impossible situation and their relationship was suffering because of it. Sophie's mother had hinted that perhaps she should get a place of her own, sooner rather than later, and Sophie was devastated by this. She had no wish to live alone or with her boyfriend. She wanted to live at home with her mother's help and guidance at hand.

The midwife asked her if she had confided any of this to her health visitor, community midwife or general practitioner and she said she had not. When asked why not she said: 'They didn't ask me the questions.' The midwife contacted the family nurse and health visitor and asked for help for Sophie and James and a plan was made to see them both in one week to discuss the issues further.

Case study 4.3

The midwife received a phone call from a school nurse asking if a young girl named Sarah had been booked at the hospital, or whether she had attended for termination of pregnancy. The midwife had no knowledge of the girl and asked for more details. The school nurse said Sarah had confided in her weeks ago that she was pregnant and that she planned to have a termination. Sarah had not attended for termination, therefore the midwife suggested that the school nurse see her and ask her if she was still pregnant.

Questions and discussion points

- Which recommendations can be implemented within midwifery services to increase continuity of care for pregnant teenagers?
- Why is the provision of a specialist midwife for teenagers likely to be more effective in terms of communication with outside agencies?
- Which recommendations can be implemented within midwifery services for pregnant teenagers to reduce the incidence of non-attendance for antenatal care?
- Which components of a specialist service for young women aged under 20 are effective in improving outcomes?

Action taken by the midwife

The staff had a genuine interest and non-judgemental attitude towards pregnant teenagers, enabling a solution to be found which suited all involved. Sensitivity to the needs of teenagers and their families enables everyone to feel confident when making plans for the future. The next day the nurse informed the midwife that Sarah was still pregnant, but was adamant that she could not tell her mother or anyone else in her family as she felt the burden of the pregnancy would be too much for her mother to bear.

The school nurse asked if a joint visit could be arranged with the midwife to meet Sarah at school and help to resolve this situation. This was arranged and the meeting was held in a private room within the school. As well as being terrified of what her mother would do or say, Sarah was also full of remorse and sadness because she felt that she had let her mother down. Sarah knew that her mother (a single parent) had a constant struggle to make ends meet financially and was genuinely worried about how they could 'afford' a new baby in the family. The midwife suggested that Sarah write a note to her mum, or send her a text message and stay out of the house until she had calmed down. Sarah thought she could not tell her mother this way. To make matters more urgent, Sarah was already feeling movements and on palpation seemed to be between 22 and 24 weeks' gestation. Sarah felt there was no one she could confide in and she was certain she wanted to continue with the pregnancy. Her boyfriend, who was the baby's father, was also aged 15 and had told her he would support her as best he could.

After a long discussion, Sarah gave permission for the midwife and school nurse to visit her mother that morning (while Sarah was in school) and tell her about the pregnancy. After the initial shock, Sarah's mother went straight to the school to comfort her daughter and offer her support. This relationship is continuing to remain positive. The bond between mother and daughter seems to have strengthened and both are looking forward to welcoming the new baby into the family.

Section 2
Care of women of advanced age

Alison Cooke and Carol Bedwell

Introduction

The trend for advanced maternal age at first birth has steadily increased over the past two decades (Office for National Statistics, 2010). Although the birth rate dropped slightly in 2009 for the first time since 2001, it continued to rise for those aged over 35 years (Office for National Statistics, 2010). Live births to women over 40 have nearly trebled from 9717 in 1990 to 27 731 in 2010 (Office for National Statistics, 2011a). These figures are in contrast to the decreasing trend in prevalence of births to those under the age of 20, and the static trend for those in the 20–24 age group (*Figure 4.1*: Office for National Statistics, 2011a).

The existing evidence base suggests that women over the age of 35 are at risk of poorer obstetric and neonatal outcomes compared to younger women aged 20–34 years. In particular, outcomes such as caesarean section, preterm delivery, stillbirth, low birth weight, and chromosomal abnormalities have all been suggested as affecting more women over the age of 35 (Gilbert et al, 1999; Forrester and Merz, 2003; Cleary-Goldman et al, 2005; Reddy et al, 2006). These possible outcomes

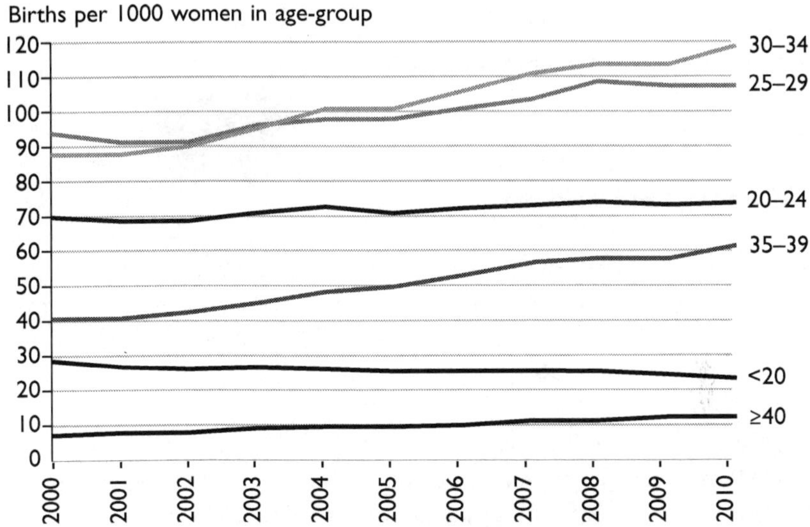

Figure 4.1. Age-specific fertility rates, England and Wales, 2000–2010. (Office for National Statistics, 2011.)

will begin to place a time/resource burden on midwives and other maternity health professionals as the demographic of their caseload gradually shifts towards an older population and consequently a more high risk group.

Current antenatal guidelines suggest that women over the age of 40 years should receive additional care (National Institute for Health and Clinical Excellence, 2008). These guidelines do not define exactly what additional care should be given and as a result varied pathways are likely to be developed by individual maternity service providers and commissioners. This may result in disparity, in which some maternity care providers may include these women in 'normal' low risk midwifery-led care whilst others may include them in high risk consultant-led care. The lack of comprehensive guidance, coupled with conflicting research evidence, can give rise to difficulties for health professionals in determining a plan of care for older mothers. Furthermore, the inconsistent definitions used in clinical practice, Government policy and research of what constitutes 'advanced' maternal age add to the confusion. Research studies have used varying definitions of advanced maternal age from age 30 and upwards to age 50, with age 35 being the most commonly used (Royal College of Obstetricians and Gynaecologists, 2009).

This section focuses on the issues facing health professionals in providing antenatal and intrapartum care to older pregnant women, guidance on care provision and the need for more specialist care pathways.

Antenatal care

NICE Antenatal Care Guidelines

The Antenatal Care Guidelines introduced by NICE in 2003, and updated in 2008, were intended to provide clear guidance on routine care to be provided in pregnancy. However, they did not specifically offer guidance for care of those women who were high risk.

> *The guideline covers recommendations on baseline clinical care for all pregnant women. It does not offer information on the additional care that some women will require. Pregnant women with the following conditions usually require care that is additional to that detailed in this guideline: higher risk of developing complications, for example, women aged 40 and older.*
>
> (NICE, 2008: 48. Clinical guideline 62 appendix C)

The NICE guidance leaves the definition of 'additional care' open to local interpretation. There are therefore likely to be inconsistencies in provision of care for older women across different healthcare trusts. Furthermore, the guidance suggests that only women over the age of 40 require additional care, although there is some evidence that risks may occur earlier; age 35 being the age most commonly agreed as the beginning of age-related increased obstetric risk (Salihu et al, 2003; Cleary-Goldman et al, 2005; Treacy et al, 2006). Currently, however, women in the 35 to 39 age group fall within the standard care remit of the NICE antenatal guidance, without further acknowledgement of age-related risks.

Early antenatal care: The booking visit

Thorough history taking is important to enable the midwife to complete an accurate risk assessment. The appointment will also reveal if the woman has faced infertility issues or has any underlying medical conditions that may impact on her pregnancy. Many older women may require fertility treatment in order to become pregnant; in 2010 58.4% of IVF treatments were to women age 35 or over (Human Fertilisation and Embryology Authority, 2011; see also *Chapter 2,* Section 2). It is important that midwives are aware of the pre-conception history and anticipate that the woman may experience increased anxiety about her pregnancy (Hjelmstedt et al, 2003). It can be difficult for women to discuss personal matters within a short consultation period on which the focus is often physical wellbeing. In order to provide appropriate care to meet possible psychological needs it is important to build up a relationship with the woman. These women may particularly benefit from models of care that allow for continuity of provider.

Antenatal assessment and management of risks

Midwives and other health professionals are likely to be caring for an increasing population of older mothers. It is important that they are aware of any risk factors associated with age that may affect the pregnancy or its outcome. The NICE Antenatal Care Guidelines (2008) assist members of the maternity service to provide consistent care and appropriate referral when deviation from a normal healthy pregnancy is recognised. See *Case study 4.4*.

At the booking interview, the midwife completes a risk assessment of the woman. The outcome of the assessment will determine whether a woman is advised to book for midwifery-led care (low risk) or consultant-led care (high risk). There is disparity between NHS trusts with regard to risk assessment proformas, particularly in relation to maternal age. In some trusts, a woman of advanced age with no other risk factors is classified as 'low risk' and receives midwifery-led care. However, in others, age alone may exclude the woman from midwifery-led care; depending on whether maternal age over 35 or 40 years is considered high risk.

It can be difficult for health professionals to determine whether a woman of advanced age should be cared for in a high or low risk environment, given the absence of robust evidence and lack of consistent clinical guidance. Advancing age is associated with increased risk of medical conditions, such as diabetes and hypertension (Salihu et al, 2003; Yancik et al, 2007). Obesity is also more prevalent as age increases (Rennie and Jebb, 2005; Low et al, 2009). The risk to these women may therefore be as a result of the underlying conditions rather than age *per se*.

The most recent maternal mortality report (Centre for Maternal and Child Enquiries, 2011) identified a marked increase in maternal death rates for older women; the death rate doubled from 9.2 per 100000 for women aged 30–34 years to 18.8 per 100000 for women aged 35–39 years, and further to 29.2 per 100000 for women aged 40 and over. Advanced maternal age is not suggested as a cause

Case study 4.4

You are presented with a 40-year-old primigravida, Angie, for antenatal booking. Her BMI is 36, she smokes 10 cigarettes a day, and has no significant medical history. She has conceived on her second cycle of IVF and has a confirmed singleton pregnancy. Her gestation is confirmed on dating scan to be 10 weeks +2 days. She appears anxious.

Questions and discussion points

- What would be your plan of care?
- What risk assessment have you made? Why have you made that assessment?
- If you have decided that Angie is high risk, is this because of age or because of another aspect of Angie's history?
- Do you feel that some of the factors mentioned are 'red herrings'? If there were no mention of raised BMI and smoking, would this woman still be considered high risk?
- Would your care be different if Angie was multiparous?

Implications for practice

Many women who present for maternity care at an advanced maternal age may be obese and may smoke. They may also have existing medical conditions that are age-related. Obesity can be age-related too. Obesity and smoking are known health risks and have a known adverse effect on pregnancy and childbirth. Existing medical conditions such as diabetes also incur an increased risk in pregnancy and childbirth. Is age *per se* the risk factor? Or is it the age-related underlying conditions that create the risk? As the literature often does not control for confounding variables it is easy to see the dilemma that health professionals face in making the risk assessment, and consequently why there are no standardised UK guidelines for care of this population of women. It highlights the importance of the need for further research to provide a strong evidence base for the development of national guidelines.

of death, however, only a common characteristic amongst those women who died from various direct or indirect causes.

It is also important to understand that older primigravid and multigravid women may have different needs. Multiparous women are not generally considered to be at the same level of risk for all obstetric outcomes, particularly if they have an uncomplicated obstetric history (Luke and Brown, 2007; Lisonkova et al, 2010; Wang et al, 2011). However, they may still be at risk of age-related conditions such as diabetes and hypertension. Hence, it is important to provide women with individually-tailored care. This may involve arranging attendance at specialist clinics, or a higher frequency of hospital or consultant visits.

Current evidence suggests that advanced maternal age is associated with increased incidence of poor pregnancy outcomes, such as chromosomal abnormalities and stillbirth (Fretts et al, 1995; Andersen et al, 2000; Bateman and Simpson, 2006). It is important for health professionals to be aware of this increased risk and be vigilant in assessments of fetal wellbeing, particularly in late pregnancy. In practical terms, this may mean extra antenatal appointments, increased fetal monitoring, and increased frequency of visits to the hospital rather than in the community.

Women themselves do not appear to be aware of all of the associated risks of delayed childbearing. The risks that women seemed aware of, in both a meta-synthesis (Cooke et al, 2010) and a UK qualitative study (Cooke et al, 2011), were infertility and chromosomal abnormalities (specifically Down's syndrome). They were unaware of other risks and some suggested that age alone should not be a risk factor (Saxell, 1996; Cooke et al, 2010, 2011).

While most women of advanced age will have healthy pregnancies and normal outcomes, health professionals need to be aware of the specific risks. These should underpin the rationale for the initial and ongoing risk assessment during pregnancy. It is also important that health professionals are able to discuss risks sensitively with women, without causing undue anxiety. This is important in empowering women with the knowledge to participate fully in informed decision making regarding their care. In relation to provision of care, older women should be cared for according to the NICE Antenatal Care Guidelines (2008) unless a complication that requires specific monitoring, such as hypertension or diabetes, is evident.

Antenatal screening

The UK National Screening Committee has produced a care pathway to assist antenatal services to provide appropriate care and referral (National Screening Committee, 2009a). The screening pathway, which is summarised in *Table 4.1*, has no separate pathway for women of advanced maternal age. Antenatal screening, which is provided through blood tests and ultrasound scans, is discussed at the booking interview so that women may make an informed decision about whether

Table 4.1. Summary of UK National Screening Committee Care Pathway (all age groups)		
When? (Approximate gestation)	*What is tested?*	*How is it tested?*
8–14 weeks	Dating scan	Ultrasound scan
10 weeks	Haemoglobin Group and antibodies Rhesus factor Syphilis Hepatitis B Rubella susceptibility HIV Sickle cell and thalassaemia	Blood test
11–14 weeks	Nuchal translucency test 1st trimester Down's syndrome	Blood test and ultrasound scan
15–20 weeks	2nd trimester Down's syndrome	Blood test
18–21 weeks	Detailed anomaly scan	Ultrasound scan

or not to proceed with it. It is not mandatory; women have a choice and may decline some or all screening or diagnostic tests.

Although antenatal screening considers many different issues such as infection and neural tube defects, for women over the age of 35 years there is a known increased risk of chromosomal anomalies (Forrester and Merz, 2003). Antenatal screening provides all women with an option to find out their risk for having a baby with a chromosomal abnormality. Screening can occur in either the first or second trimester of pregnancy. The current best practice is for this screening test to take place in the first trimester, between 10 and 14 weeks' gestation. This early screening test, known as the nuchal translucency (NT) test consists of both a blood test, which measures the serum markers of pregnancy-associated plasma protein A (PAPP-A) and human chorionic gonadotrophin (hCG) hormone, and an ultrasound scan, which measures the NT space at the back of the fetal neck. This is the preferred pathway and is now recommended over second trimester screening, known as the quadruple test, taken at 14–20 weeks. This is a blood test which takes into account four biochemical markers to determine the risk of chromosomal anomaly: alpha fetoprotein (AFP), B-hCG, oestriol and inhibin. The quadruple test remains the recommended screening pathway for those women who book for maternity care too late to have the NT screening (about 15% of the pregnant population; National Screening Committee, 2011). Screening is not a diagnostic test but may provide women with information regarding their risk status which may then inform their decision making regarding further diagnostic testing such as chorionic villus sampling (CVS) or amniocentesis. Women having the earlier, first trimester screening may opt for CVS which can be performed between 10 and 14 weeks of pregnancy. This has the advantage of early diagnosis of Down's syndrome, although there is also a risk of miscarriage of 1–2% with this procedure (Royal College of Obstetricians and Gynaecologists, 2010). Women opting for second trimester screening are likely to be offered amniocentesis at 15–18 weeks of pregnancy should the screening result place them in a high risk category. Women aged up to 35 years may be more likely to opt for diagnostic testing when faced with the risk tables indicating that having a baby with Down's syndrome is shown to increase significantly for their age group; for example, at age 20 years the risk of Down's syndrome is 1:1500 women, compared to 1:270 at the age 35 and 1:100 at age 40 (NHS, 2004).

Age-related risk may still be a shock to some women even if they were aware of an increased risk of chromosomal anomaly. It is important that health professionals bear this in mind when advising women about the screening available. For a woman who may have struggled to conceive in the first place, the risk of miscarriage (1% following amniocentesis and 1–2% following CVS; Royal College of Obstetricians and Gynaecologists, 2010) may make this decision hard to make. The earlier NT screening may mean more recourse to CVS. Although CVS has a higher risk of miscarriage, if a decision to terminate the pregnancy was made by the woman, this could be done through dilatation and curettage. A decision to terminate following amniocentesis would require going into labour and giving birth, which a woman may feel is more traumatic. Health professionals need to be sensitive to a woman's needs and expectations. It is important to be aware that some women may not consider screening appropriate if they are sure they would not proceed with diagnostic testing if a positive screening result was determined, due to the increased risk of miscarriage. Parents and health professionals are sometimes unaware that there is a choice with regard to screening tests (Skirton and Barr, 2010).

Studies are currently investigating the potential of non-invasive prenatal diagnosis (NIPD) and cell-free fetal DNA (cffDNA) using maternal blood tests alone. These have the potential to reduce the number of women needing to undergo CVS or amniocentesis and will also provide earlier detection since the blood sample is taken at approximately five weeks' gestation. This would provide parents with a longer period of time to make informed decisions about the pregnancy or provide the possibility of terminating the pregnancy at an earlier gestation (National Screening Committee, 2009b).

Ongoing antenatal care: Specialist services

Maternal age is likely to represent a continuum of risk. However, current evidence supports the NICE guidelines (2008) that identify maternal age over 40 with a clinically significant increase in poor pregnancy outcome. Hence, consultant-led care, with midwifery input, may be advocated for women over 40. It may be appropriate for women aged 35–39, without other risk factors, to access midwifery-led care. Dependent on individual NHS trust policies, women of advanced age may be cared for under any of these patterns of care. Whatever the care package, it is important that the plan is individualised to meet the women's needs. Women with additional medical or obstetric risk factors such as pre-existing or previous pregnancy-induced hypertension or diabetes, should be referred to an obstetrician. These women may require specialist care, possibly within specialist clinics, but should continue to receive midwifery input. This may result in additional appointments, or may form part of the scheduled appointments as per NICE guidance (2008).

For many women, attendance at a high risk clinic can result in the provision of care by a doctor rather than a midwife. When providing high risk care, health professionals may lose sight of a woman's expectations of normality (Berg, 2002). Women may attend their first antenatal appointment with hopes and aspirations for a normal pregnancy, labour and birth (Saxell, 1996). They may desire this regardless of their risk status (Saxell, 1996). It is essential that women are aware of, and understand, any risk factors they may have, so that they may make informed choices throughout their pregnancy and birth. This will require collaborative working of the multidisciplinary team including both midwives and obstetricians. A plan of care can be put into place to meet the woman's needs. A meeting between the obstetric team and the supervisor of midwives could be arranged to determine how best a woman's desires for antenatal care and birth could be achieved. For example, a home birth may be achievable for a woman who is considered high risk providing the consultant and supervisor of midwives have agreed a plan with the woman with regard to the conditions under which she would need to be transferred to the obstetric unit from home. This should be well documented in the maternity notes for the benefit of the midwife providing intrapartum care.

It is clear that women of advanced maternal age require appropriate services to meet their needs with regard to their increased risk of poorer obstetric and neonatal outcomes. Whether these are best provided by a specialist service is open to debate. Many hospital trusts provide a variety of specialist clinics, including services for women with pregnancies complicated by hypertension, diabetes or fetal growth restriction (FGR). There are often specialist clinics for obesity or smoking cessation. Where necessary and appropriate, women of advanced maternal age should be referred to these services. It may not be appropriate to provide a specialist service for women of advanced maternal age *per se* without strong evidence to support it. However, it is vital that all women gain midwifery support during their pregnancy and for those receiving high risk care, the provision of midwifery input is vital. This could be achieved simply by ensuring that a woman attending specialist hospital clinics is given extra appointments to meet her named midwife/midwives in the community.

Given the risk factors that have been associated with advanced maternal age, it is important that health professionals are vigilant in detecting these in pregnancy. Guidelines for the management of hypertension in pregnancy (NICE, 2010b) suggest that primigravid women aged 40 years and over are at increased risk of pre-eclampsia and should be prescribed 75mg aspirin daily from 12 weeks' gestation. Age is also an additional risk factor for pre-eclampsia for those with gestational hypertension (first incidence after 20 weeks' gestation without significant proteinuria). Current evidence also suggests that advanced maternal age is associated with an increased incidence of late *in utero* fetal death (see *Chapter 3*, Section 1). In the absence of congenital abnormality, 50% of stillbirths and neonatal deaths are associated with FGR (Gardosi et al, 2005). FGR is recognised to be a preventable cause of perinatal death, providing there are effective strategies in place to detect and monitor the at risk fetus (Perinatal Institute, 2007).

A standard antenatal appointment should include blood pressure monitoring, urinalysis, measurement of symphysis fundal height (preferably plotting recordings on a customised growth chart), in addition to general assessment of maternal and fetal wellbeing. If any deviation from normal is evident, such as hypertension, suspected FGR, indicated by the symphysis fundal height being lower than the predicted curve on a customised growth chart, or reduced fetal movements, then the midwife should refer the woman to the hospital for obstetric review. Further investigations such as blood pressure profiling, blood tests to screen for pre-eclampsia, ultrasound assessment of fetal growth and liquor volume, and Doppler and cardiotocograph monitoring may be ordered. This may involve attending an antenatal clinic, antenatal or labour ward, scan department, day unit or maternity triage. Depending on the outcome of any further investigations, the woman may be discharged or given additional, more frequent appointments to monitor progress. If the deviation from normal resolves, a woman may be transferred back to midwifery-led care. If not, the woman may find that the majority of future appointments are with the obstetric team.

Later antenatal care: Preparation for birth/parent education

In some areas, specialist parent education or antenatal classes are provided for young parents, because they are perceived to experience discomfort in attending a class with older women (Sykes, 2006). Figures released by the National Childbirth Trust reveal 30% of women attending their classes are aged over 35 (Newburn et al, 2011); it is unknown how many women over the age of 35 attend NHS-provided classes. In addition, older mothers are more likely to access internet sources to gain further information about pregnancy and birth (Redshaw and Heikkila, 2010). However, the quality and relevance of the information available via the internet may be questionable. Although consideration may be given to providing tailored classes, since women themselves may not consider age to be an issue, offering specific age-related classes might only serve to stigmatise them.

The assumption is that older mothers have high incomes and are educated and articulate (Doughty, 2009). However, this may not always be the case and it is important that all women are offered equity of access to parent education classes (NICE, 2008). The National Perinatal Epidemiology Unit maternity survey report (Redshaw and Heikkila, 2010) noted that women aged over 40 are less likely to have been offered access to parent education classes than those aged 19 years or below (65% compared with 80%). Reasons for this may include the perception that older women do not need the same level of support, or are more likely to be motivated to access such services themselves. However, parent education classes are unable to cover all aspects of care and it is important that women with additional risk factors have their needs addressed. This may be more appropriately carried out as part of antenatal care, on a one-to-one basis with the woman's midwife. Therefore, it is important that health professionals understand any additional care needs the woman may have and have the time to discuss these with her.

Intrapartum care

Place of birth

Government policy (Department of Health, 2007) advocates that women should be offered choice in determining place of birth. However, for women classified as high risk, the most appropriate setting for birth may be an obstetric unit (NICE, 2007). This will particularly affect older women with pre-existing conditions which place them in a high risk category. The increased risk of late gestation stillbirth with advancing maternal age has generated debate on whether interventions should be offered to improve outcomes. Reddy et al (2006) studied the risk of stillbirth in women ≥35 years compared to those <35. At 37–41 weeks' gestation the relative risk of stillbirth was 1.32 (95%CI 1.22–1.43) increasing to 1.88 (95%CI 1.64–2.16) for women ≥40, with the peak stillbirth risk at 41 weeks (*Figure 4.2*). These data support policies that advocate induction of labour or increased electronic fetal monitoring from 37–38 weeks due to the rise in risk at that gestation (Bateman and Simpson, 2006; Reddy et al, 2006; Hoffman et al, 2007). As yet there have been no randomised controlled trials to assess the effectiveness and acceptability of early induction of labour in older women. Until sufficient evidence is available, decisions regarding induction of labour should be taken by a senior obstetrician with due regard to the woman's wishes and other risk factors. This is an area in which guidance is currently being considered by the Royal College of Obstetricians and Gynaecologists (2011).

The increased risk of stillbirth associated with maternal age, along with increased pregnancy surveillance and monitoring, is likely to lead to a greater number of older women being offered induction of labour. An obstetric unit may be the most suitable setting for many, but not all, older women. Many older women approach labour and birth with a degree of preparedness and expectation and, therefore, may be more likely to be aware of their options for place of birth. Recent research into birthplace indicated that more women in the 35–39 age group planned to give birth at home than in an obstetric-led unit (Birthplace in England Collaborative Group, 2011). Figures from the Office for National Statistics (2011b) also indicate that the highest proportion of home births occur in the 35–39 age group (*Figure 4.3*). It is important to note, however, that these figures also include unplanned births.

Women require optimum care and support in their choice of place of birth and labour and birth itself, regardless of age. Despite the documented risks related to age, older women choose and succeed in having births, without intervention, at home. Appropriate planning, in conjunction with the woman, taking into account

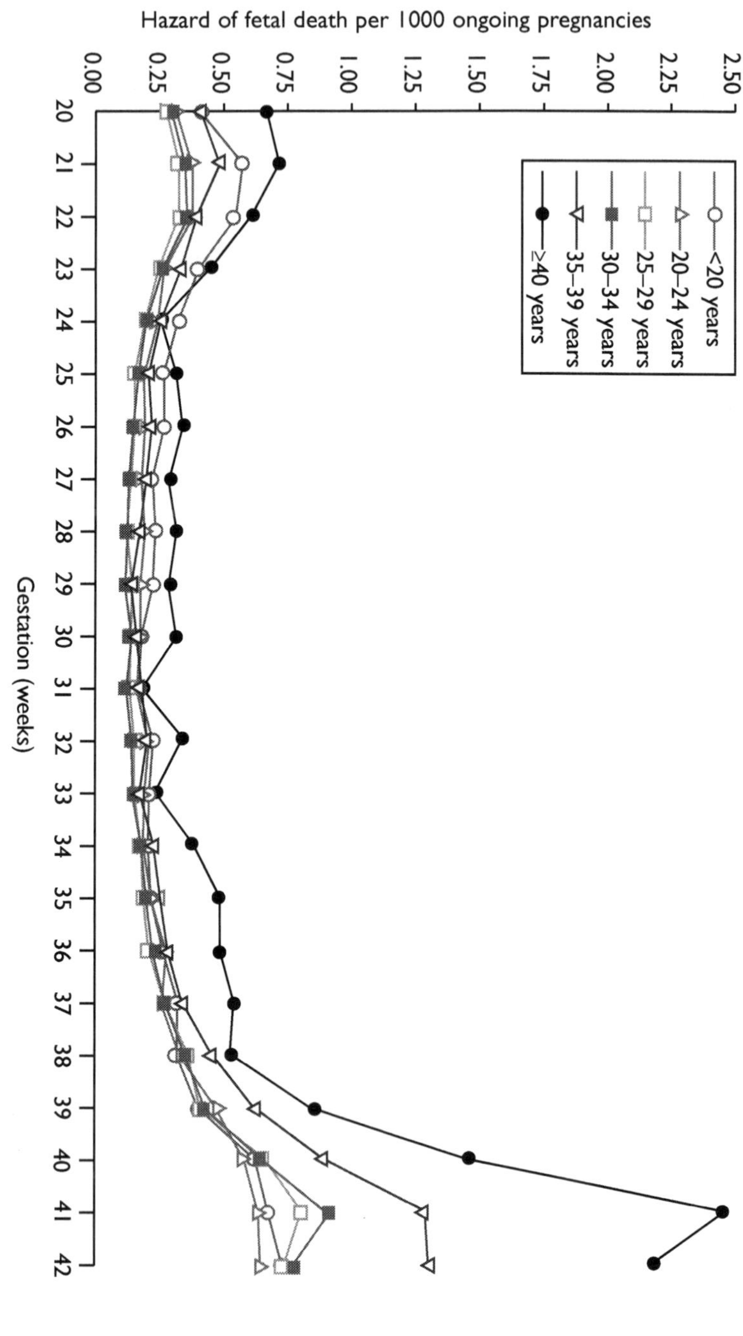

Figure 4.2. Hazard (risk) of stillbirth for singleton births without congenital anomalies by gestational age, 2001–2002. Reprinted from American Journal of Obstetrics and Gynecology, 195(3), Reddy UM, Chia-Wen K and Willinger M, Maternal age and the risk of stillbirth throughout pregnancy in the United States, Pp 764–70, with permission from Elsevier.

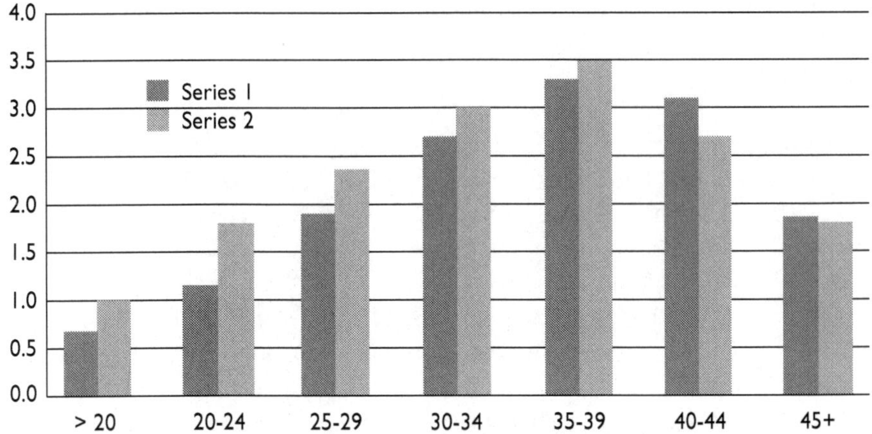

Figure 4.3. Home birth and maternal age, England and Wales, 2000–2010. (Source: Office for National Statistics (2011b). Contains public sector information licensed under the Open Government Licence v1.0.)

risk factors to determine the most suitable birth setting and approach to birth is paramount both for optimum outcomes and the best experience for the woman.

Care in labour

Intrapartum care should be focused towards the individual needs of the woman and her family. Ideally, options for care will be discussed prior to labour. The writing of a birth plan should be encouraged and may enable women to focus on normality, a positive mental attitude, and confidence in their ability to give birth (Kaufman, 2007). It will also provide health professionals with the opportunity to discuss plans for labour in advance. Although older women may be more likely to require induction or acceleration of labour, where possible, they should be offered the same opportunities in labour as any other woman, including options for analgesia, mobility and positions for birth.

Health professionals themselves need to be mindful of the potential increased risks associated with advanced maternal age, including the well-documented increased risks of caesarean section and stillbirth for women who delay childbearing (Gilbert et al, 1999; Cleary-Goldman et al, 2005; Reddy et al, 2006). Other age-related conditions or multiple pregnancies, which may have occurred as a result of fertility treatment, all require extra care in labour. Women with complex needs or risk factors need appropriate multidisciplinary care, provided in an obstetric unit. However, as with all women, they should be encouraged to engage in decision making throughout, and health professionals should aim to make the experience as positive as possible.

The perception of the older mother is often one of a stable and supported individual. However, it is important for care givers to be aware that this may not be the case and some older mothers may lack peer or family support (Cooke et al, 2010). Support in labour is known to improve outcomes and lead to less intervention (Hodnett et al, 2011), hence, it is important that this area is not overlooked for this group of women.

Whether classified as high or low risk, all women should be offered choice and be involved in decisions. As far as possible normality should be promoted, but it is important to recognise that complications may occur and care in labour will need to reflect such complications.

Conclusion

In this section, we have addressed the issues facing midwives and other health professionals caring for women of advanced maternal age. In reality, until clear guidelines are provided, the majority of these women will be cared for within the existing maternity care framework, until such time as they deviate from 'normal'. Many women in this group will present with other issues, such as obesity, smoking or existing medical conditions. Individualised care planning should ensure that women can access the specialist services necessary for them. Health professionals must be sensitive to a woman's needs, as they may not have any perception of being at additional risk in pregnancy and childbirth.

Further research may assist with the development of improved guidelines towards the care of women of advanced maternal age. There may be a need for specialist care pathways or clinics in view of the increasing trend for women being older at first birth. It would be preferable if this were standardised best practice across UK maternity units. There is a dearth of research, audit and evaluation of any specialist care provided, although this may in fact exist in 'pockets' of the UK. A survey of maternity units could assess current care provision and provide a basis for evaluation of any specialist services. Quality services could then be rolled out across the UK, or serve as a basis for guiding future research to establish evidence of best practice for this population. Women over the age of 35 years are a rapidly increasing childbearing group and more robust research is required to enable us to be clear on what additional care, if any, is required for them. Until then, individualised care should be our focus with sensitivity to women's expectations.

Discussion questions

- How do we overcome the difficulty in informing women of the risks when we, as health professionals, are not absolutely confident in the evidence base ourselves?
- Is it too late to be informing women about the risks when they are already pregnant? When would be the best time to inform them?

References

Andersen A, Wohlfahrt J, Christens P, Olsen J, Melbye M (2000) Maternal age and fetal loss: Population based register linkage study. *British Medical Journal* **320**: 1708–12

Bateman B, Simpson L (2006) Higher rate of stillbirth at the extremes of reproductive age: A large nationwide sample of deliveries in the United States. *American Journal of Obstetrics and Gynecology* **194**: 840–5

Berg M (2002) *Genuine caring in caring for the genuine. Childbearing and high risk as experienced by women and midwives*. Comprehensive Summaries of Uppsala Dissertations from the Faculty of Medicine. Acta Universitatis Uppsaliensis, Sweden

Birthplace in England Collaborative Group (2011) Perinatal and maternal outcomes by planned place of birth for healthy women with low risk pregnancies: The Birthplace in England National Prospective Cohort Study. *British Medical Journal* **343**: d7400 doi: 10.1136/British Medical Journal.d7400

Bolling K, Grant C, Hamlyn B, Thornton A (2007) *Infant Feeding Survey 2005*. The Information Centre for Health and Social Care. Available from: www.ic.nhs.uk

Bonell C, Allen E, Strange V, Copas A, Oakley A, Johnson A, Stephenson J (2005) The effect of dislike of school on risk of teenage pregnancy: Testing of hypotheses using longitudinal data from a randomised trial of sex education. *Journal of Epidemiology and Community Health* **59**: 223–30

Bristol Booking Survey (1983) *A Publication of European Collaborative for Child Health, Teenage Mothers*. Powage Press, University of Bristol

Burchett H, Seeley A (2003) *Good enough to eat: The diet of pregnant teenagers*. Maternity Alliance/Food Commission. London. www.maternityalliance.org.uk

Centre for Maternal and Child Enquiries (2011) Saving Mothers' Lives: Reviewing maternal deaths to make motherhood safer: 2006-2008. *British Journal of Obstetrics and Gynaecology* **118**: 1–203

Cleary-Goldman J, Malone F, Vidaver J et al (2005) Impact of maternal age on obstetric outcome. *Obstetrics and Gynecology* **105**: 983–90

Clemmens D (2001) The relationship between social support and adolescent mothers' interactions with their infants: A Meta-Analysis. *Journal of Obstetric, Gynaecology and Neonatal Nursing* **30**: 410–20

Cooke A, Mills TA, Lavender T (2010) 'Informed and uninformed decision making' – Women's reasoning, experiences and perceptions with regard to advanced maternal age and delayed childbearing: A meta-synthesis. *International Journal of Nursing Studies* **47**: 1317–29

Cooke A, Mills TA, Lavender T (2011) Advanced maternal age: Delayed childbearing is rarely a conscious choice. A qualitative study of women's views and experiences. *International Journal of Nursing Studies* **49**: 30–9

Corbin T (2004) Mortality in children under 8. *Health Statistics Quarterly* **24**: 30–7

Dallison J, Lobstein T (1995) *Poor expectations: Poverty and undernourishment in pregnancy*: Maternity Alliance/NCH Action for Children, London

Department for Children, Schools and Families (2008) *Teenage parents: Who cares? A guide to commissioning and delivering maternity services for young parents*. HMSO, London

Department of Health (1992) *The health of the nation: A strategy for health in England.* HMSO, London

Department of Health (2001) *Infant feeding initiative.* HMSO, London

Department of Health (2004) *National service framework for children, young people and maternity services*. Available from: www. dh.gov.uk/en/Publicationsandstatistics/Publications/

Department of Health (2007) *Maternity matters*. HMSO, London

Department of Health, Department for Children, Schools and Families (2007) *Teenage Parents Next Steps: Guidance for Local Authorities and Primary Care Trusts*. HMSO, London

Dewan N, Brabin B, Wood L, Drammond S, Cooper C (2003) The effects of smoking on birth weight for gestational age curves in teenage and adult primigravidae. *Public Health* **117**: 31–5

Dewan N, Wood L, Maxwell S, Cooper C, Brabin B (2002) Breastfeeding knowledge and attitudes of teenage mothers in Liverpool. *Journal of Human Nutrition and Dietetics* **15**: 33–7

Doughty S (2009) *Number of babies born to mothers over 40 has doubled in a decade*. Available from: www.dailymail.co.uk/news/article-1185782/Number-babies-born-mothers-40-DOUBLED-decade.html [Accessed: 1 May 2012]

Dyson L, Renfrew M, McFadden A, McCormick F, Herbert G, Thomas J (2006) *Promotion of breastfeeding initiation and duration*. National Institute for Health and Clinical Excellence Evidence into practice briefing. Available from: www.nice.org.uk

Edwards G (2000) Teenage pregnancies: A baseline audit. *The Practising Midwife* **3**(5): 10–13

Ermisch J, Pevalin D (2003) *Does a "teen birth" have longer-term impact on the moth-*

er? Evidence from the 1970 British Cohort Study. Institute for Economic and Social Research, Working Papers, University of Essex

Forrester M, Merz R (2003) Maternal age-specific Down syndrome rates by maternal race/ethnicity Hawaii: 1986–2000. *Birth Defects Research* **67**: 635–9

Fraser AM, Brocker JE, Ward RH (1995) Association of young maternal age with adverse reproductive outcomes. *New England Journal of Medicine* **332**: 1113–7

Fretts R, Schmittdiel J, McLean F, Usher R, Goldman M (1995) Increased maternal age and the risk of fetal death. *New England Journal of Medicine* **333**: 953–7

Furey A (2004) Are support and parenting programmes of value for teenage parents? Who should provide them and what are the main goals? *Public Health* **118**(4): 262–7

Gardosi J, Kady SM, McGeown P, Francis A, Tonks A (2005) Classification of stillbirth by relevant condition at death (ReCoDe): Population based cohort study. *British Medical Journal* **331**: 1113–7

Gilbert W, Nesbitt T, Danielsen B (1999) Childbearing beyond age 40: Pregnancy outcome in 24,032 cases. *Obstetrics and Gynecology* **93**: 9–14

Goyder E, Blank L, Peters J (2003) *Supporting teenage parents: The potential contribution. Research Report 8, University of Sheffield*. Available from: http://ndcevaluation.adc.shu. ac.uk/ndcevaluation/Reports.asp

Hedger ML, Scholl TO, Belsky DH (1989) Weight gain during pregnancy and pregnancy outcome. *New Jersey Obstetrics and Gynaecology* **74**: 1

Hjelmstedt A, Widstrom AM, Wramsby H, Collins A (2003) Patterns of emotional responses to pregnancy, experience of pregnancy and attitudes to parenthood among IVF couples: A longitudinal study. *Journal of Psychosomatic Obstetrics and Gynecology* **24**: 153–62

Hodnett ED, Gates S, Hofmeyr GJ, Sakala C, Weston J (2011) Continuous support for women during childbirth. *Cochrane Database of Systematic Reviews 2*: Art. No.: CD003766. DOI: 10.1002/14651858.CD003766.pub3

Hoffman M, Jeffers S, Carter S, et al (2007) Pregnancy at or beyond age 40 years is associated with an increased risk of fetal death and other adverse outcomes. *American Journal of Obstetrics and Gynecology* **196**: e11–13

Human Fertilisation and Embryology Authority (2011) *Fertility treatment in 2010*. Available from: www.hfea.gov.uk/docs/2011-11-16_-_Annual_Register_Figures_Report_final.pdf (Accessed 4th January 2012)

Kaufman T (2007) Evolution of the birth plan. *Journal of Perinatal Education* **16**, 37–52.

Keirnan K (1995) *Transition to parenthood: Young mothers, young fathers – associated factors and later life experiences*. LSE Discussion paper WSP/113

Konje K, Palmer A, Watson D, Hay M, Imrie I (1992) Early teenage pregnancies in Hull. *British Journal of Obstetrics and Gynaecology* **99**(12): 969–73

Lavender T, Thompson S, Wood L (2005) Supporting teenage mothers with breastfeeding guardians. *British Journal of Midwifery* **13**(6): 354–9

Lisonkova S, Janssen PA, Sheps SB, Lee SK, Dahlgren L (2010) The effect of maternal age on adverse birth outcomes: Does parity matter? *Journal of Obstetrics and Gynaecology Canada* **32**: 541–8

Low S, Chin MC, Deurenberg-Yap M (2009) Review on epidemic of obesity. *Annals Academy of Medicine* **38**: 57–65

Luke B, Brown MB (2007) Elevated risks of pregnancy complications and adverse outcomes with increasing maternal age. *Human Reproduction* **22**: 1264–72

Mayhew E, Bradshaw J (2005) Mothers, babies and the risks of poverty. *Poverty* **121**: 13–6

Miller HS, Lesser KB, Reed KL (1996) Adolescence and very low birth weight infants: A disproportionate association. *Obstetrics and Gynaecology* **87**: 83–8

National Health Service (2004) *National Down's syndrome screening programme for England: A handbook for staff.* UK National Screening Committee, London

National Institute for Health and Clinical Excellence (2007) *Intrapartum care: Care of healthy women and their bBabies during childbirth. Clinical Guideline 55.* National Collaborating Centre for Women's and Children's Health, London

National Institute for Health and Clinical Excellence (2008) *Antenatal care: Routine care for the healthy pregnant woman.* Available from: www.nice.org.uk/guidance/CG62. NICE, London

National Institute for Health and Clinical Excellence (2010a) *Pregnancy and Complex Social Factors. NICE clinical guideline 110,* www.nice.org.uk/guidance/CG110

National Institute for Health and Clinical Excellence (2010b) *Hypertension in pregnancy: The management of hypertensive disorders during pregnancy.* NICE, London

National Institute for Health and Clinical Excellence (2011) *Caesarean section clinical guideline CG132.* NICE, London

National Screening Committee (2009a) *18+0 to 20+6 weeks fetal anomaly screening care pathway.* NHS, Exeter

National Screening Committee (2009b) *Information for women in non-invasive prenatal diagnosis (NIPD) and cell-free fetal DNA (cffDNA).* NHS, Exeter

National Screening Committee (2011) *Screening for Down's syndrome: UK NSC Policy recommendations 2011–2014: Model of Best Practice'.* NHS, Exeter

Newburn M, Muller C, Taylor S (2011) *Preparing for birth and parenthood: Report on first-time mothers and fathers attending NCT antenatal courses.* NCT, London

Office for National Statistics (2010) *Live births.* Available from: www.statistics.gov.uk/CCI/nugget.asp?ID=369 [Accessed: 8th September 2010]

Office for National Statistics (2011a) *Births and deaths in England and Wales, 2010.* Statistical Bulletin. ONS, Newport

Office for National Statistics (2011b) *Characteristics of birth 2, England and Wales, 2010. Statistical Bulletin.* ONS, Newport

Perinatal Institute (2007) *Confidential enquiry into stillbirths with fetal growth restric-*

tion. Perinatal Institute, Birmingham

Reddy U, Ko C, Willinger M (2006) Maternal age and the risk of stillbirth throughout pregnancy in the United States. *American Journal of Obstetrics and Gynecology* **195**: 764–70

Redshaw M, Heikkila K (2010) *Delivered with care: A national survey of women's experience of maternity care 2010*. National Perinatal Epidemiology Unit, Oxford

Rennie KL, Jebb SA (2005) Prevalence of obesity in Great Britain. *Obesity Reviews* **6**: 11–12

Royal College of Obstetricians and Gynaecologists (2009) *Reproductive ageing*. RCOG Press, London

Royal College of Obstetricians and Gynaecologists (2010) *Amniocentesis and chorionic villus sampling green-top guideline no.8*. RCOG Press, London

Royal College of Obstetricians and Gynaecologists (2011) *Induction of labour at term in older mothers. Consultation document.* Available from: http://www.rcog.org.uk/womens-health/consultation-documents [Accessed: 2 January 2012]

Russell JK (1988) Early teenage pregnancy. *Maternal and Child Health* **13**: 2

Salihu H, Shumpert N, Slay M, Kirby R, Alexander G (2003) Childbearing beyond maternal age 50 and fetal outcomes in the United States. *Obstetrics and Gynecology* **102**: 1006–14

Saxell L (1996) Nulliparous women's perception of the risk of pregnancy after age 35. *Health and Canadian Society* **4**: 367–87

Simms M, Smith C (1984) Late comers to medical and ante-natal care. *Midwife, Health Visitor and Community Nurse* **20**: 192–200

Simms M, Smith C (1986) *Teenage mothers and their partners. DHSS Research Report 15*. HMSO, London

Skirton H, Barr O (2010) Antenatal screening and informed choice: A cross-sectional survey of parents and professionals. *Midwifery* **26**: 596–602

Smith T (1993) Influence of socioeconomic factors on attaining targets for reducing teenage pregnancies. *British Medical Journal* **306**: 1232–5

Swann C, Bowe K, McCormick G, Kosmin M (2003) *Teenage pregnancy and parenthood: A review of reviews*. Health Development Agency, London

Sykes S (2006) *Qualitative evaluation study of teenage antenatal classes and an evaluation review of teenage parent support groups provided in Croydon*. Croydon PCT, London

Teenage Pregnancy Unit, Department of Health Nursing and Midwifery Policy, Royal College of Midwives (2004). *Teenage parents: Who cares? A guide to commissioning and delivering maternity services for young parents*. RCM, London

Treacy A, Robson M, O'Herlihy C (2006) Dystocia increases with advancing maternal age. *American Journal of Obstetrics and Gynecology* **195**: 760–63

Wang Y, Tanbo T, Abyholm T, Henriksen T (2011) The impact of advanced maternal age and parity on obstetric and perinatal outcomes in singleton gestations. *Archives of Gynecology and Obstetrics* **284**: 31–7

Wellings K, Nanchahal K, MacDowall W, McManus S, Erens B, Mercer CH, Johnson AM, Copas AJ, Korovessis C, Fenton KA, Field J (2001) Sexual behaviour in Britain: Early heterosexual experience. *Lancet* **358**: 1834–50

Wiggins M, Oakley A, Sawtell M, Austerberry H, Clemens F, Elbourne D (2005) *Teenage parenthood and social exclusion: A multi-method study.* Social Science Research Unit Report, Institute of Education, University of London

Yancik R, Ershler W, Satariano W, Hazzard W, Cohen H, Ferrucci L (2007) Report of the National Institute on Aging Task Force on Comorbidity. *Journals of Gerontology Series A* **62**: 275–80

Chapter 5

Effective postnatal care

Debra Bick

Introduction

Large observational studies undertaken in the UK and Australia, published over 20 years ago, were the first to highlight the impact of pregnancy and birth on a woman's physical and psychological wellbeing (MacArthur et al, 1991; Glazener et al, 1995; Brown and Lumley, 1998). Many women experienced health problems including backache, urinary and faecal incontinence, perineal pain and depression, symptoms of which were infrequently reported by the women and not identified by the attending healthcare professional. Furthermore, for some women health problems experienced following birth persisted well beyond the 6–8 week postnatal period when women are routinely discharged from maternity care in the UK (Bick and MacArthur, 1995).

A number of randomised trials have since assessed the outcome of interventions aimed at promoting the early identification and management of maternal morbidity, including early GP consultation within a week of the birth compared with the 6–8 week consultation (Gunn et al, 1998), use of community-based maternity support workers (Morrell et al, 2000) and protocol-based, extended midwifery-led postnatal care in the community (MacArthur et al, 2002, 2003). Trials have assessed the benefit of the interventions compared with current care, including measures of physical and psychological health and wellbeing and use of health service resources. To date, the only trial that found a significant difference in maternal health was that led by MacArthur and colleagues (2002, 2003) which found a statistically significant difference in maternal mental health outcomes at 4 and 12 months postpartum. This was also one of the few trials that revised routine care as opposed to assessing the impact of an 'addition' to routine care.

One of the main criticisms is that current models of routine postnatal care do not identify maternal health needs. The focus of midwifery care is on specific physical signs of birth recovery, and the current organisation and timing of NHS maternity services does not enable flexibility of care to meet individual women's health needs, which may benefit from a longer period of contact with the midwife. Although the use of medical interventions during labour and birth, such as caesarean section, have increased, and women with more complex health needs are becoming pregnant (Information Centre, 2011; Centre for Maternal and Child Enquiries, 2011), the number of days women spend as inpatients on the postnatal ward has decreased. The number of contacts a woman may receive from her midwife at home has also decreased (Care Quality Commission, 2010).

Maternity service policy has recognised the important role effective and timely postnatal care could play in the promotion of shorter and longer-term maternal and infant health and wellbeing, especially among more vulnerable women (Department of Health, 2004, 2007; NICE, 2006). However, a recent survey of first-time mothers, which looked for evidence of change in practice and service provision in line with National Institute for Health and Clinical Excellence (NICE) (2006) guidance, indicated that many women did not receive the care recommended in the guidance to promote recovery (Bhavani and Newburn, 2010). Recent changes to routine postnatal care services, driven by demands to reduce resource use, such as the introduction of postnatal clinics in some parts of England, have not been subject to formal evaluation, and the impact on women's recovery is as yet unknown.

As well as acknowledgement that all women require effective postnatal care because of widespread and persistent morbidity (NICE, 2006), it is increasingly recognised that some groups of women in developed countries, such as the UK, may be more susceptible to severe maternal morbidity, and in some cases mortality, as a consequence of developing conditions such as eclampsia, amniotic fluid embolism, haemorrhage and stroke (Centre for Maternal and Child Enquiries, 2011; Kayem et al, 2011). As majority of maternal deaths occur after the birth (Centre for Maternal and Child Enquiries, 2011), there is a clear need for effective, planned postnatal care.

Cohort and case control studies have identified that one of the major contributing factors to severe maternal and infant morbidity and mortality is younger and older maternal age. However, age may be just one of a number of inter-related risk factors for poor maternal outcome; other factors include a woman's social and demographic characteristics, her health behaviours, such as smoking and diet, and how many years of full-time education she received. When assessing the evidence, it is important to consider if all potential confounding factors have been considered. In addition to morbidity and mortality issues, maternal age and other associated factors could also influence decisions about method of infant feeding and the choice and use of contraception (Information Centre, 2011; NICE, 2005).

The implications of younger and older maternal age for the provision of effective postnatal care are the focus of this chapter, which commences with an overview of age-associated risk factors for poor pregnancy outcome. It is important that midwives and other members of the healthcare team are aware of the need for vigilance for women who may be more vulnerable to poor outcome. As definitions of 'older' and 'younger' age vary across studies and reports, this chapter will refer to the definitions used by study authors. Reference is made to the guideline for routine postnatal care published by NICE (2006), as this presents evidence-based recommendations for promotion and implementation of effective postnatal care.

Severe postnatal morbidity and mortality

The work of the Confidential Enquiries into Maternal Deaths has made an important contribution to our understanding of risk factors for maternal mortality. As UK maternal mortality rates are very low (Centre for Maternal and Child Enquiries, 2011), work is now in progress to inform our awareness of risk factors for severe maternal morbidity, evidence of which will support revisions to promote high quality maternity care. The UK Obstetric Surveillance System (UKOSS) collates data to inform a rolling programme of studies that focus on pre-specified serious, potentially life-threatening health conditions from every consultant-led maternity unit in the UK (Knight et al, 2005).

A recent paper from the UKOSS team reported on a national cohort study of data collated from 2003 to 2009 on women who died and women who survived five specific maternal conditions: eclampsia, antenatal pulmonary embolism, acute fatty liver of pregnancy, amniotic fluid embolism and antenatal cerebral stroke. Data on women who died were obtained from the Centre for Maternal and Child Enquiries team. Of 476 women who were identified and survived and 100 who died from these conditions, maternal death was associated with older maternal age (35 years and above), black ethnicity and being unemployed or employed in manual or routine occupations. There was also an association with obesity.

Appropriate statistical analyses were undertaken, with the incidence of maternal mortality and severe maternal morbidity, and ratio of survivors to deaths calculated for each condition with 95% confidence intervals and logistic regression analyses used to investigate potential factors underlying the morbidity and mortality data. With respect to older maternal age, of note, the team found that the risk of progressing from severe morbidity to death in their sample was not associated with any co-existing disease as reported in previous studies (Lewis, 2007; Schutte et al, 2010). The UKOSS study authors postulate that older maternal age confers a physical disadvantage, with older women lacking physiological robustness to react to pregnancy pathology. Older women and their medical teams may not appreciate this risk and women postponing childbirth need to be made aware of it (Kayem et al, 2011). During the period 2006–2009 the highest maternal mortality rates were among women aged 40 and over (29.2 per 100 000 maternities; Centre for Maternal and Child Enquiries, 2011).

Teenage pregnancy has become a major public health issue in the UK, which has the highest teenage pregnancy rate in Europe, with one study showing that 70% of teenage pregnancies are unplanned (Social Exclusion Unit, 1999). It is difficult to quantify the precise effect of a teenage pregnancy on birth outcomes, given the number of potential confounding factors that may be associated, including lower socioeconomic status and access to education, and health behaviours such as smoking and alcohol intake. In contrast to older women, younger women have the lowest maternal mortality rate, at 8.6 per 100 000 maternities during 2006–2008 (Centre for Maternal and Child Enquiries, 2011). While teenage pregnancy may be a positive experience for women, particularly in the later teen years (Bonnell, 2004), one of the main concerns is the adverse impact it can have on health and social outcomes for the woman and her child.

According to observational and case control studies, poorer pregnancy outcomes identified to be more common among younger women, include pre-eclampsia and eclampsia, sepsis, premature birth, infant death and congenital anomalies (Rees et al, 1996; Phipps et al, 2002; Paranjothy et al, 2009; Acosta et al, 2012). However, some study findings are conflicting due to the associated influence of adverse social circumstances. A study that considered severe maternal morbidity in Canada using routine hospital data from 2003 to 2007 (Joseph et al, 2010) reported a severe maternal morbidity rate of 13.8 per 1000 births, with rates higher among births to older women, women having their first babies and women who had a multiple birth.

A recent large retrospective cohort study from one centre in Canada, which included data on over 9000 women giving birth to their first babies between 2001 and 2007, compared adverse pregnancy outcomes by age group (Shrim et al, 2011). Among the women, 250 (2.6%) were aged 19 years or younger, the remaining women were aged from 20 to 39 years of age. Teenage women were more likely to have a premature birth, and higher rates of extreme prematurity. Their babies were more likely to have a lower birth weight, and were more likely to be admitted for neonatal care. Logistic regression analysis showed a significant association between younger maternal age and at least one adverse pregnancy outcome.

Sepsis as a cause of maternal mortality is rare in developed countries, although deaths from sepsis have doubled over the past 20 years in the UK (Centre for Maternal and Child Enquiries, 2011). A population-based case-control study of maternal sepsis undertaken in the North of Scotland NHS region found, after controlling for mode of birth and sociodemographic and clinical factors, that maternal age of 25 years or younger (odds ratio 5.15, 95%, CI 2.43–10.90), obesity (odds ratio 2.12, 95%, CI 1.14–3.89) and operative vaginal delivery (odds ratio 2.20, 95%, CI 1.02–4.87) were significant predictors of sepsis (Acosta et al, 2012). The researchers recommended that these risk factors should be considered when planning clinical care.

One of the issues for women in the younger age group is the potential to not seek appropriate and timely care. Barriers to seeking timely and appropriate antenatal care by women aged 20 years and younger included, for example, the way women perceived they were treated by health staff, personal reasons, and barriers reported by service providers (NICE, 2010a). Little is known of younger women's use of postnatal services, with studies relevant to care in the UK in the main addressing interventions to assess impact on health behaviours in the postnatal period. These are referred to in the following sections where appropriate.

Commonly reported morbidity

Physical morbidity

Some of the more commonly experienced physical health problems women report are associated with maternal age, although again caution is needed given the number of confounding factors that could influence outcomes. This is particularly important with respect to parity. Primiparity is highly associated with younger maternal age and with a number of commonly experienced health problems but consideration would have to be given to establish if age or parity was the independent predictor of the outcome of interest. Midwives need to be aware of risks to younger and older women in order to support planning of effective postnatal care.

Backache is a very common symptom experienced both during and after pregnancy. Some studies report a prevalence of around 50%, with symptoms persisting for months or even years after giving birth (MacArthur et al, 1991; Brown and Lumley, 1998). With high rates of backache reported in the general population, it is difficult to attribute the extent to which pregnancy can be the primary cause. More women having their first babies are likely to opt for epidural analgesia and reports from earlier studies found an association between epidurals and new onset backache (MacArthur et al, 1990; Brown and Lumley, 1998), with a potential association suggested with a woman's stressed posture during labour. More recent studies have documented the use of lower concentrations of local anaesthetic with an opiate to produce a less dense 'block', enabling women to mobilise in labour. A two-centre randomised controlled trial comparing traditional epidural block with two different low dose 'mobile' epidurals found no significant difference in backache reported by women starting within six weeks of birth and lasting longer than three months in either mobile technique (COMET Study Group, 2001).

Stress urinary incontinence is a symptom more likely to be reported by multiparous women (MacArthur et al, 2006), with some evidence of a higher prevalence among older women (Glazener et al, 2006). Other factors associated with this symptom include higher body mass index (Viktrup et al, 2006) and heavier infant birthweight (Hojberg et al, 1999). Epidemiological and urodynamic studies have reported that caesarean section is less likely to be associated with urinary incontinence (Glazener et al, 2006; Viktrup et al, 2006), although longitudinal studies have reported a prevalence of this symptom of around 15% among women who only ever had a caesarean birth (MacArthur et al, 2006).

Large observational and pathophysiological studies generally concur that the two main factors associated with the occurrence of faecal incontinence and occult anal sphincter defects are instrumental delivery and third/fourth degree tear (Bick et al, 2008). Parity may be associated with both of these outcomes, with women having a first baby more likely to have instrumental birth. Donnelly et al (1998), in a study of sphincter damage in 124 primiparous women, found instrumental delivery to be associated with an 8.1-fold (odds ratio 95%, CI 2.7–24.0) risk of anal sphincter injury and a 7.2-fold (odds ratio 95%, CI 2.8–18.6) risk of symptoms (urgency, and faecal and flatus incontinence). Abramowitz et al (2000) found forceps delivery to be an independent predictor of damage (odds ratio 12, 95% CI 4–20). Most studies are too small to be conclusive about the relative effects of instrumental delivery by forceps or by vacuum extraction. MacArthur et al, (2001), in a large study of 4214 women at three months postpartum, separately examined associations with each of the instruments and found that relative to spontaneous vaginal delivery, forceps delivery was independently associated with faecal incontinence (odds ratio 1.94, 95% CI 1.30–1.29), but vacuum extraction was not (odds ratio 1.26, 95% CI 0.77–2.07).

The main risk factors for perineal pain and dyspareunia identified in studies relate to mode of vaginal birth, perineal trauma and primiparity (Glazener, 1997; Signorello et al, 2001; Buhling et al, 2006). These factors are all clearly highly inter-related so again, caution is needed when interpreting findings. Perineal pain is commonly experienced, with around 70% of women who have a vaginal birth sustaining perineal trauma which requires suturing (Bick et al, 2008). Brown and Lumley (1998) contacted 1336 women 6–7 months postpartum, in a cross-sectional study of all births occurring over two weeks within a region in Australia, and found that for 21% a painful perineum had been a problem at some time since the birth. The proportion who still had this at 6–7 months was not given. A prospective cohort study from Canada which examined differences in perineal pain relative to the type of trauma sustained among 444 women who had a vaginal birth, found that overall 92% reported pain on the first day after the birth, and 61% reported pain on the seventh day (MacArthur and MacArthur, 2004); 7% had perineal pain when questioned about this six weeks after the birth. Superficial dyspareunia was experienced by two-thirds of primiparous women who had resumed sexual intercourse within three months of birth in a study of women who gave birth at one London maternity unit, half of whom reported symptoms six months post-birth (Barrett et al, 2000). Reports of an association between dyspareunia and extent of perineal trauma are conflicting. Andrews et al (2008), in a prospective study of 241 women having their first vaginal birth, reported that 40% had resumed sexual activity within seven weeks of the birth, with no association with type or extent of perineal trauma. In contrast, an earlier study by Larsson et al (1991) of over 2000 births reported a 5% reduction in dyspareunia when women who had spontaneous tears were compared with women who had an episiotomy.

The rate of caesarean births in the UK has increased dramatically over the past 20 years, from 11.3% in 1990 to 24.8% in 2010 (Information Centre, 2011), with evidence that women pregnant at an older age are at a higher risk of a caesarean birth (Luke and Brown, 2007). Caesarean section birth has a strong association with endometritis and surgical site infection (Lamont et al, 2011), with a reported five to 20-fold increased risk of infection compared to vaginal birth, although this varies by timing of assessment and definition of infection (Hager et al, 2004). There is no standard definition of endometritis, with national guidance for postnatal care within the NHS (NICE, 2006) referring to the World Health Organization (2006) definition of symptoms, including a temperature over 38°C and any of the following: feeling very weak, abdominal tenderness, foul-smelling lochia, profuse lochia, uterus not well contracted, lower abdominal pain, or history of heavy vaginal bleeding. Surgical site infection data are poorly collated as many women will develop infection after postnatal hospital discharge, with information based on audit which may not be comprehensive. There is no universally agreed definition of surgical site infection following caesarean section, with rates reported in a UK population study of 11 units in the East Midlands of England of around 14% (range between units 2–17%), the majority of which occurred following postnatal hospital discharge (Ward et al, 2008). Risk factors were indentified in this study as high body mass index, younger maternal age, blood loss, method of wound closure and emergency caesarean section birth.

Headaches are commonly reported in the general population and among women who have recently given birth, as shown in large observational studies. Glazener et al (1995), in a longitudinal study, examined maternal postnatal morbidity in over 1200 women, who comprised a 20% random sample of deliveries in the Grampian region of Scotland between June 1990 and May 1991. All women were given a questionnaire whilst on the postnatal ward, a postal questionnaire at eight weeks, and half of the women were sent another questionnaire 12–18 months after the birth. Headaches of any duration, including new and recurrent symptoms, were reported by 14% of women whilst in hospital, by 22% between hospital discharge and eight weeks and by 15% after this. Symptoms may persist, as shown in a large cluster randomised controlled trial of a new model of midwifery-led postnatal care which focused on identification and management of common health problems up to three months post-birth (MacArthur et al, 2002). When women were followed up at 12 months post-birth, headaches were reported by 26% overall, with no difference in symptoms between the intervention and control groups (MacArthur et al, 2003). As with the study by Glazener et al (1995), women were not asked to distinguish between new and ongoing symptoms. It is likely that in the majority of cases, women were experiencing tension headaches, or migraine.

Midwives should be alert to the reporting of the onset of a severe headache within the first week of birth associated with a woman moving from a supine to a postural position as this could indicate a possible post-dural puncture headache, where the pain is triggered by traction on the meninges. The incidence of accidental dural puncture is low; a recent survey of anaesthetists responsible for obstetric services in the five Nordic countries (*n* = 153) reported an incidence of around 1%. The epidural rate was defined in the study as the number of epidurals for labour divided by total number of births, and accidental dural puncture defined as the number of punctures divided by the number of epidurals for labour. Only hospitals in Iceland recorded full data on the incidence of accidental dural puncture. A review of 10 years of use of combined spinal anaesthesia for elective caesarean section birth in one English unit reported a puncture rate of 0.7%, with a 52% incidence of severe post-dural puncture headache (Sadashivaiah and McLure, 2009).

Psychological morbidity

Women may experience a range of mental health disorders during and after pregnancy, including anxiety disorders, depression and postnatal psychotic disorders (NICE, 2007). Some disorders may be self-limiting, while others may be long-term and, if not managed effectively, could impact on longer-term outcomes for the woman and her family. When considering incidence and prevalence of mental health disorders in a perinatal population, care has to be given to the timing and method of assessment, as many studies have reported findings from self-assessment of symptoms. Care should also be taken to ensure 'depression' is not used as a 'catch all' phrase to describe women's mental health, as this could be misleading, and other serious illness could be misdiagnosed as a consequence (Lewis and Drife, 2004).

Risk factors for perinatal mental health disorders have been considered in a large number of studies. Factors examined include maternal and obstetric characteristics, previous psychiatric history, personal relationships and hormonal influences. A systematic review of potential risks for mental disorders (Robertson et al, 2004) presented risk factors in order of magnitude of effect size. These were depression or anxiety during pregnancy, life events, poor social support, previous history of depression, neuroticism and poor marital relationships. Low socioeconomic status and obstetric factors had small effect sizes. A more recent large prospective study from Australia of antenatal risk factors for postnatal depression, which collated the antenatal Edinburgh Postnatal Depression Scale (EPDS) scores of over 35 000 women and postnatal EPDS scores of over 22 000 women, found that scores of greater than 12 on the scale postnatally were independently predicted by antenatal depression, together with a prior history of depression and a low level of partner support (Milgrom et al, 2008). With respect to maternal age, social factors identified as having a negative impact on perinatal mental health outcomes are more likely to be experienced by younger women, and particular consideration has to be given to the content of the maternity care they receive (NICE 2010a).

Supporting optimal physical and psychological recovery from birth

All women should receive effective and timely postnatal care to promote recovery from birth. This should be informed by a plan of care tailored to the individual needs of the woman (NICE, 2006). Care should reflect particular support needs including those that may be required by older and younger women based on evidence as highlighted above. As referred to earlier, several trials of interventions implemented in the postnatal period that aimed to reduce maternal morbidity and improve experiences and views of care have been completed (Gunn et al, 1998; Morrell et al, 2000; Reid et al, 2000; MacArthur et al, 2002, 2003). However, only the large cluster randomised controlled trial by MacArthur et al (2002, 2003) found clinical and cost-effective differences between the trial intervention group and the usual care group.

The trial by MacArthur et al (2002, 2003) assessed the development and implementation of a model of midwifery-led community-based postnatal care. General practices ('clusters') were randomised to the intervention or the control group, and midwives attached to the practice were asked to continue to provide usual care or the new model of care, depending on which group the practice had been allocated to. With respect to the intervention, all women were to be visited by their midwife up to 28 days post-delivery, with visits planned on individual need. To support identification of common morbidity, the midwife was asked to administer a checklist at 10 days and 28 days to help identify health needs, and had evidence-based guidelines to support management of any problems reported. A final home visit was to be arranged between 10 and 12 weeks post-delivery, at which point the woman was discharged from the maternity services; this visit replaced the routine GP 6–8 week check.

Primary trial outcomes included composite physical and mental health scores of the SF36, a general health measure, and EPDS scores as assessed at 4 and 12 months' post-birth. There was a statistically significant difference in mental health outcomes at 4 and 12 months, with women who received the new model of care less likely to have higher scores on both measures. The effect size persisted to 12 months indicating that the new model could enhance longer-term mental health. GP consultations during the first year post-birth were also reduced among women in the intervention group. Women's views of care were more positive among those who received the new model of care, including feeling better able to talk to their midwife about health problems, or did not differ from women in the control group.

Since this trial was published, several important policy reports and guidelines have made a series of recommendations for the content and planning of effective postnatal care, including the *National service framework for children, young people and maternity services* (Department of Health, 2004), the NICE postnatal care guideline (NICE, 2006), *Maternity matters* (Department of Health, 2007), NICE guidance on antenatal and postnatal mental health (NICE, 2007), and complex social factors in pregnancy (NICE, 2010b).

In 2006, the NICE guideline for routine care of women and their babies was published with recommendations to be implemented by the NHS maternity services in England and Wales. This included specific guidance for the content of care to be implemented within the first 24 hours, the first two weeks and up to eight weeks postpartum. The guideline provided recommendations for maternal and infant health and wellbeing, including signs and symptoms of severe morbidity, and infant feeding. The following sections refer to the NICE guidance to support effective care.

Planning effective postnatal care

NICE (2006) recommends that all women should have an individualised postnatal care plan, tailored to their individual needs, and that development of the care plan should be commenced antenatally (see *Box 5.1*). This could be particularly

Box 5.1. Planning postnatal contacts

NICE recommends a documented, individualised postnatal care plan, developed with the woman, ideally in the antenatal period or as soon as possible after birth to include:

- Relevant factors from the antenatal, intrapartum and immediate postnatal period
- Details of the healthcare professionals involved in her care and that of her baby including roles and contact details
- Plans for the postnatal period

This should be reviewed at each postnatal contact. There should be local protocols about written communication, in particular about the transfer of care between clinical sectors and healthcare professionals. These protocols should be audited.

Women should be offered relevant and timely information to enable them to promote their own and their babies' health and wellbeing and to recognise and respond to problems.

At the first postnatal contact, women should be advised of the signs and symptoms of potentially life-threatening conditions and to contact their healthcare professional immediately, or call for emergency help, if any signs and symptoms occur.

NICE (2006: 5)

important for women in the younger and older age groups who could benefit from care planned across the continuum of antenatal, intrapartum and postnatal care. This could include opportunities to implement interventions which may reduce poor outcome (for example, antenatal perineal massage for women having their first baby which is associated with reduced incidence of perineal trauma; Beckman and Garrett, 2006) and early identification of postnatal morbidity. The care plan should be updated at every contact, including asking women about vaginal loss, their emotional health, healing of any perineal trauma and emotional attachment with their baby.

Younger women, who may not have the same level of social support as older women, may require help in accessing such support following the birth of their baby. They may also require interventions to promote positive health behaviours, such as quitting or reducing smoking; women under 20 are five times more likely to smoke during pregnancy than women aged 35 years or over (45% vs. 9%) (British Market Research Bureau, 2007), and interventions to promote smoking cessation need to be implemented after birth in addition to during the antenatal period. Women at both age continuums are also likely to benefit from advice on weight gain before, during and after pregnancy, particularly for those who have a BMI of 30 and over at the commencement of their pregnancy (NICE, 2010b). There is evidence that maternal obesity and weight retention after birth are associated with social deprivation (Heslehurst et al, 2010).

There is limited evidence of the extent to which antenatal commencement of postnatal plans is being implemented. A recent study of a systems and process approach to redesigning inpatient postnatal care as part of a quality improvement initiative introduced new postnatal records (Beake et al, 2010) which were offered to women at 28 weeks' gestation and included information for women on planning their postnatal care (Bick et al, 2011a). A post-intervention survey of the midwives who implemented a revision to care found that most felt care was better planned and more appropriate to meet maternal needs. However, concerns were raised that in some cases midwives were not completing postnatal documentation, adding to the workload of the midwife who made the subsequent contact with the woman (Bick et al, 2011a).

Care within the first 24 hours

In addition to commencing the postnatal element of a woman's care plan, NICE (2006) guidance recommends that information on signs and symptoms of severe morbidity is offered to all women within 24 hours of birth. For younger and older women, given evidence of the risk of severe morbidity and mortality as referred to earlier in this chapter, it is very important that midwives adhere to this guidance. The conditions for which signs and symptoms of onset are described were based on the most commonly reported reasons that women died following birth during the triennium 2003–2005, which included post-partum haemorrhage, genital tract sepsis, pre-eclampsia, eclampsia and thrombosis (Lewis, 2007). The most recent triennial report into maternal mortality published in 2011, and covering the period 2006–2008, reported that sepsis was the most common cause of direct maternal death in the period following birth (Centre for Maternal and Child Enquiries, 2011). Most deaths occurred in the postnatal period, were often preceded by a sore throat or other upper respiratory infection, and had a clear seasonal pattern. An associated factor was women of black and minority ethnic origin, and more than half of deaths followed caesarean section. Deaths from sepsis were very rare, with a maternal mortality rate of 1.13/100000 maternities; nevertheless, the important message for midwifery care is that sepsis is not a symptom confined to the history books. The need for increased awareness of sepsis among women and health professionals, for promotion of good hygiene and for constant vigilance for signs and symptoms leading to early recognition and prompt referral, could help to save lives (Bick et al, 2011b). Midwives should promote and share NICE guidance on signs and symptoms of sepsis and other potentially life-threatening conditions with women and their partners. Age is clearly one of the factors associated with severe maternal morbidity.

Care within the first postnatal week

NICE (2006) guidance recommends that, within the first postnatal week, women should be offered information on methods and timing of resumption of contraception. This advice would appear to be particularly important for younger women, and provision of advice on contraception is an accepted component of routine postnatal care, although few studies have considered the value of this advice.

Teenage women have a higher risk of repeat pregnancy within two years of the index birth (Boardman et al, 2006) and use of contraception by younger women is likely to be inconsistent (Kelly et al, 2005). A Cochrane Library systematic review of postpartum education interventions to support contraceptive use included eight studies from developed and developing countries which compared the effectiveness of interventions commenced within one month of the birth (Lopez et al, 2010). None of the included trials was from the UK. Of the eight trials, four assessed short-term counselling (defined as one to two contacts where contraception was discussed), although one of these four trials included insufficient data and one was too small to be of value to the review. The other trials looked at longer-term home or clinic-based programmes with multiple contacts.

The review found that two of the short-term interventions, which were provided during the inpatient postnatal stay, increased contraceptive use compared to no intervention. Three of the studies that considered longer-term interventions were also more effective than usual care, with one trial resulting in more effective contraceptive use and two leading to fewer repeat pregnancies in teenagers. The need for healthcare providers to develop and evaluate programmes relevant for their local populations was recommended by the reviewers (Lopez et al, 2010).

A recent prospective cohort study from Australia that followed a population of teenage mothers (aged 18 years and younger) at three month intervals over a two year period reported that use of long-acting contraceptives was associated with reduced repeat pregnancy (Lewis et al, 2010). Within 24 months postpartum, 138 women (94% of the initial 147 participants) had resumed sex. Of these, 41 (30%) did so without using contraception. Most (106; 77%) had resumed sex by three months postpartum, with 55 women (52%) initially having no contraceptive cover. Of the 147 women, 49 (33%) had a repeat pregnancy within the two years. Sexual intercourse was independently significantly associated with using oral contraception (odds ratio 2.83, 95% CI 1.38–5.82); living with the birth father (odds ratio 8.43, 95% CI 5.12–13.86); intending to become pregnant (odds ratio 3.20, 95% CI, 1.53–6.65); smoking marijuana (odds ratio 2.60, 95% CI 1.38–4.79); and using alcohol (odds ratio 1.93, 95% CI 1.17–3.20). Use of long-acting contraceptives was associated with reduced odds of repeat pregnancy (odds ratio 0.27, 95% CI 0.12–0.62), while teenagers who used an oral contraceptive had a similar risk of a repeat pregnancy compared with those using barrier methods or no contraception.

NICE (2006) also refers to the importance of encouraging maternal/paternal infant attachment during the first week post-birth and the offer of group-based parent education. These interventions may be particularly important for young women. A Cochrane Library review was undertaken of interventions that assessed individual and group-based parenting programmes for improving psychosocial outcomes for teenage parents and their children (Barlow et al, 2011). Eight studies of interventions offered to young parents aged 20 years or younger were included with data on over 500 women. Two of the studies were undertaken in Canada and six were from the USA. The methodological quality of the included studies was poor with significant clinical heterogeneity. Meta analyses were possible for nine study comparisons, the results of four of these analyses showing improved outcomes as a result of parenting programmes on outcomes of parent responsiveness to their child and parent–child interaction. Given the risk of bias from the included studies, the reviewers recommend further research is undertaken.

The Department for Children, Schools and Families/Department of Health guidance (2009) emphasises the need to engage young fathers in the care of their infants, through provision of maternity services that are easily accessible and welcoming, that treat young people with respect and that protect their confidentiality. The principles in *Box 5.2*, although not specific to the postnatal period, are important core principles of care following birth.

First two to eight weeks

NICE (2006) recommends that in the first two to eight weeks following the birth, women should be advised on signs and symptoms of common health problems. As discussed earlier, few women will report health problems, emphasising the importance of the role of the midwife in asking women about their problems at each contact. NICE guidance (2006) provides evidence-based recommendations for management, including timing of referral if symptoms persist. A recent study which aimed to enhance outcomes of routine in-patient postnatal care, revised the

Box 5.2. Principles of a young-people friendly maternity service

- An environment welcoming to young women and young men
- Easily accessible services
- Clarity about confidentiality and child protection
- Young people are treated with respect
- An empowering approach
- Accessible information that meets both parents' needs
- Young fathers' value is openly acknowledged
- Strong referral links with relevant agencies
- Effective support to both young parents to prevent second unplanned pregnancies
- Staff trained to work with young women and men

Department for Children, Schools and Families/
Department of Health (2009: 11–12)

routine postnatal records to prompt midwives to use a symptom checklist (Bick et al, 2011a). From the evidence described previously, maternal age is a potential risk factor for commonly experienced morbidity and the content of care should be planned appropriately. In addition to asking women about physical health, NICE (2006) also highlights the need to ask about emotional and psychological wellbeing at each contact.

Infant feeding

Breastfeeding is recommended because of the numerous health benefits for the infant and mother. Breast milk has been shown to protect babies against infection, including gastrointestinal and urinary infection (Howie et al, 1990; Marild et al, 2004), and juvenile onset insulin-dependent diabetes mellitus (Sadauskaite-Kuehne et al, 2004). There is also evidence to indicate that breastfed babies have a reduced risk of becoming obese (Fewtrell et al, 2004). Maternal benefits include reduced risk of premenopausal breast cancer and some forms of ovarian cancer (Department of Health, 1994) and a possibility of protection against hip fractures in older age (Department of Health, 1998). In addition, breastfeeding provides unique maternal–infant contact, and ready availability of food for the baby.

Breastfeeding uptake and duration in UK populations has been considerably lower than in other European countries, with particularly low uptake amongst younger women (Bolling et al, 2007). The most recent UK infant feeding survey has reported an increase in breastfeeding uptake rate to 81% of the population compared with 76% in 2005 when the previous national survey was completed (Information Centre, 2011). Breastfeeding rates were lowest across the UK as a whole among women under the age of 20 (58%) and highest among mothers who were aged 30 and over (87%). As reported in previous infant feeding surveys, breastfeeding uptake was more likely among older women, among first time mothers and women who had been in full-time education until 18 years of age (Information Centre, 2011). Across the UK as a whole, the incidence of breastfeeding was 91% among women who left full-time education aged 18 or over compared with 75% among women who left education aged 17 or 18, and 63% among women who left when they were aged 16 years or younger (Information Centre, 2011), an increase on the 59% who breastfed in 2005 (Bolling et al, 2007; Information Centre, 2011). Interventions that may support younger women to commence and continue breastfeeding could result in improved clinical outcomes, be cost-effective and have a positive impact on public health outcomes. Observational studies from the UK and other developed countries have consistently reported that younger mothers, those from lower socioeconomic groups and of younger age when leaving full-time education are much more likely to stop breastfeeding within a few days or weeks of the birth (Bick et al, 1998, Tucker et al, 2011, Hauck et al, 2011).

Since most studies have used quantitative methods, subtle social and cultural influences that could affect decisions about infant feeding may not have been identified. A qualitative study of 21 women, which sought to improve understanding of how primiparae belonging to lower income groups decided to feed their infants, suggested that breastfeeding is a skill that needs to be learnt, particularly by women with little exposure to other breastfeeding women (Hoddinott and Pill, 1999). These authors suggest that women may benefit from an antenatal apprenticeship with a known breastfeeding mother although low rates of breastfeeding over the past two decades mean that many women may not have access within their social network to an effective role model.

In a more recent study, Hauck et al (2011) completed a cross-sectional survey to examine infant feeding practices during the hospital stay and at nine weeks post-birth in Western Australian women who registered a live birth between February and June 2006. Data obtained from 2669 women revealed a 93% (n = 2472) initiation rate of breastfeeding. More multiparous women (73.5%) were exclusively breastfeeding in hospital compared to primiparous women (65.2%), which decreased to 57.1% and 49.2%, respectively, at nine weeks. Of women who had ceased breastfeeding by nine weeks, more multiparous women (71.1%) ceased before three weeks. Reasons cited for ceasing included insufficient milk supply, infant-related reasons, pain and discomfort, and emotional reasons. Younger maternal age, primiparous women, lower maternal education levels, being offered a combination of breast milk and formula in hospital and caesarean birth were significant independent predictors of early cessation. These are reasons similar to those reported in UK population studies (Information Centre, 2011).

A systematic review of the nature of support for teenage mothers, which included seven studies, identified five types of support available: emotional, esteem, instrumental, informational and network (Hall Moran et al, 2007). Study participants seemed to find the emotional, esteem and network components of support most helpful. Support from the young women's mothers seemed to be particularly influential. The provision of continuity of care from an expert individual who is skilled in both lactation support and working with adolescents was also highly valued by breastfeeding adolescents. There was also evidence to suggest that targeted breastfeeding educational programmes, specifically designed for the adolescent learner, may be successful in improving breastfeeding initiation and continuation rates in this population. However, a question still arises about which elements of the complex package on offer were most effective

The environment of birth may also impact on a woman's decision to breastfeed. The NICE postnatal care guideline (2006) recommended that all maternity units in England and Wales introduce a structured training programme to support breastfeeding, using the WHO/UNICEF Baby Friendly Initiative (BFI) as a minimum standard (NICE, 2006). The BFI is a global initiative which was launched in 1992 to encourage maternity units to support breastfeeding through implementation of 10 steps, and was introduced into the UK in 1994. A recent narrative review was completed of structured compared with non-structured programmes to support the uptake and duration of breastfeeding in acute and primary care settings, although few studies were conducted in the UK (Beake et al, 2011). Most of the studies included in the review found a statistically significant improvement in breastfeeding initiation following introduction of a structured breastfeeding programme, although effect sizes varied. The impact on the duration of exclusive breastfeeding and duration of any breastfeeding to 6 months was also evident, although not all studies found statistically significant differences. Despite poor overall study quality, structured programmes compared with standard care positively influenced the initiation and duration of exclusive and any breastfeeding. In healthcare settings with low breastfeeding initiation and duration rates, structured programmes may have a greater benefit. This may be a way for midwives to work with younger women to support breastfeeding outcomes. However, specific community-based interventions to support an increase in breastfeeding duration have had variable success, with calls for more consideration to be given to complex systems in which policies and interventions occur (Hoddinott et al, 2010). The NICE guidelines for successful breastfeeding are shown in *Box 5.3*.

Further considerations

There continues to be limited revision to the content and timing of current postnatal care with some evidence from large surveys of service users' views that services have declined (Care Quality Commission, 2010). Given the range of morbidity reviewed in this chapter that can affect women, and the potential for improved outcomes as a consequence of effective postnatal care, it is important that midwives, managers, service providers and commissioners continue to promote the importance of this critical period of time for women and their families. There should also be acknowledgement of the role of evidence to support the content and duration of care.

Box 5.3. NICE recommendations for successful breastfeeding

- Offer additional breastfeeding support to women who have had a narcotic/ general anaesthetic, a caesarean or delayed contact with their baby
- Ensure breast pumps are available for women who have been separated from their babies and give instruction on how to use them
- If formula feeding, advise on how to prepare, store and warm formula and how to clean and sterilise bottles and teats
- Encourage unrestricted breastfeeding frequency and duration
- Reassure women about breast milk supply and help them gain confidence
- Advise women that babies will stop feeding when satisfied
- Advise women of the signs that a baby is successfully feeding:
  - swallowing is audible and visible
  - there is a sustained rhythmic suck
  - the arms and hands are relaxed
  - the mouth is moist
  - there are regular soaked/heavy nappies

NICE (2006: 37)

Discussion questions

- How can members of the multiprofessional health team ensure that the postnatal care provided meets the physical and psychological needs of vulnerable women?
- What factors do you think influence women's postnatal decisions? How do they interact with age?
- In your clinical practice, what do you do to identify and document commonly reported morbidity? Is this sufficient? If not, what could you change?

References

Abramowitz L, Sobhani I, Ganansia R et al (2000) Are sphincter defects the cause of incontinence after vaginal delivery? Results of a prospective study. *Diseases of the Colon Rectum* **43**: 590–6

Acosta CD, Bhattacharya S, Tuffnell D, Kurinczuk JJ, Knight M (2012) Maternal sepsis:

A Scottish population-based case-control study. *British Journal of Obstetrics and Gynaecology* **119**(4): 474–83

Andrews V, Thakar R, Sultan AH, Jones PW (2008) Evaluation of postpartum perineal pain and dyspareunia – A prospective study. *European Journal of Obstetrics and Gynecology and Reproductive Biology* **137**(2):152-6

Barlow J, Smailagic N, Bennett C, Huband N, Jones H, Coren E (2011) Individual and group based parenting programmes for improving psychosocial outcomes for teenage parents and their children. *Cochrane Database of Systematic Reviews* **3**: Art. No. CD002964

Barrett G, Pendry E, Peacock J, Victor C, Thakar R, Manyonda I (2000) Women's sexual health after childbirth. *British Journal of Obstetrics and Gynaecology* **107**(2): 186–95

Beake S, Pellowe C, Dykes F, Schmied V, Bick D (2011) A systematic review of structured compared with non-structured breastfeeding programmes to support the initiation and duration of exclusive breastfeeding in acute and primary healthcare settings. *Maternal and Child Nutrition* DOI: 10.1111/j.1740-8709.2011.00381 [Epub ahead of print]

Beake S, Rose V, Bick D, Weavers A, Wray J (2010) A qualitative study of women's experiences and expectations of in-patient postnatal care in one English maternity unit. *BMC Pregnancy and Birth*. Available from: http://www.biomedcentral.com/1471-2393/10/70

Beckmann MM, Garrett AJ (2006) Antenatal perineal massage for reducing perineal trauma. *Cochrane Database of Systematic Reviews* **1**: Art. No. CD005123

Bhavnani V, Newburn M (2010) *Left to your own devices: The postnatal care experiences of 1260 first-time mothers*. National Childbirth Trust: London

Bick D, Beake S, Pellowe C (2011) Maternal genital tract sepsis: Vigilance must continue to be a priority. *The Practising Midwife* **14**(4): 16–18

Bick D, MacArthur C (1995) The extent, severity and effects of health problems after childbirth. *British Journal of Midwifery* **3**: 27–30

Bick DE, MacArthur C, Lancashire R (1998) What influences the uptake and early cessation of breast feeding? *Midwifery* **14**: 242–7

Bick D, MacArthur C, Winter H (2008) *Postnatal care. Evidence and guidelines for management* (2nd edn). Churchill Livingstone, London

Bick D, Weavers A, Rose V, Wray J, Beake S (2011) Improving inpatient postnatal services: Midwives' views and perspectives of engagement in a quality improvement initiative. *BMC Health Services Research* **11**(1): 293

Boardman LA, Allsworth J, Phipps MG, Lappane KL (2006) Risk factors for unintended versus intended rapid repeat pregnancies among adolescents. *Journal of Adolescent Health* **39**: 597

Bolling K, Grant C, Hamlyn B, Thornton A (2007) *Infant feeding survey 2005*. The Information Centre, London

Bonell CP (2004) Why is teenage pregnancy conceptualised as a social problem? A review of quantitative research from the USA and UK. *Culture, Health and Sexuality* **6**: 1–18

British Market Research Bureau (2007) *Infant feeding survey 2005. A survey conducted on behalf of the Information Centre for Health and Social Care and the UK Health Departments.* Information Centre, Southport

Brown S, Lumley J (1998) Changing childbirth: Lessons from an Australian survey of 1336 women. *British Journal of Obstetrics and Gynaecology* **105**: 143–5

Buhling KJ, Schmidt S, Robinson JN, Klepp C, Siebert G, Dudenhausen JW (2006) Rate of dyspareunia after delivery in primiparae according to mode of delivery. *European Journal of Obstetrics Gynecology and Reproductive Biology* **124**(1): 42–6

Care Quality Commission (2010). Maternity services survey England 2010. Care Quality Commission, London

Centre for Maternal and Child Enquiries (2011) Saving mothers' lives: Reviewing maternal deaths to make motherhood safer – 2006–08. The eighth report of the Confidential Enquiries into Maternal Deaths in the United Kingdom. *British Journal of Obstetrics and Gynaecology* **118**(Sppl 1): 1–203

COMET Study Group (2001) Effect of low-dose mobile versus traditional epidural techniques on mode of delivery: a randomised controlled trial. *The Lancet* **358**: 19–23

Darvish B, Gupta A, Alahuhta S, et al (2011) Management of accidental dural puncture and post-dural puncture headache after labour: A Nordic survey. *Acta Anaesthesiologica Scandinavica* **55**(1): 46–53

Department for Children, Schools and Families/Department of Health (2009) *Getting maternity services right for pregnant teenagers and young fathers*. Revised Edition. Department for Children, Schools and Families, Nottingham

Department of Health (1994) *Weaning and the weaning diet.* The Stationery Office, London

Department of Health (1998) *Department of Health, Nutrition and Bone Health COMA Expert Group. Report on health and social subjects 49.* The Stationery Office, London

Department of Health (2004) T*he national service framework for children, young people and maternity services*. Department of Health, London

Department of Health (2007) *Maternity matters: Choice, access and continuity of care in a safe service*. The Stationery Office, London

Donnelly VS, Fynes M, Campbell D, Johnson H, O'Connell PR, O'Herlihy C (1998) Obstetric events leading to anal sphincter damage. *Obstetrics and Gynecology* **92**(6): 955-961

Fewtrell MS, Lucas A, Cole TJ, Wells JC (2004) Prematurity and reduced body fatness at 8-12 years of age. *American Journal of Clinical Nutrition* **80**(2): 436–40

Glazener CMA (1997) Sexual function after childbirth: Women's experiences, persistent morbidity and lack of professional recognition. *British Journal of Obstetrics and*

Gynaecology **104**: 330–5

Glazener C, Abdalla M, Stroud P, Templeton A, Russell I (1995) Postnatal maternal morbidity: Extent, causes, prevention and treatment. *British Journal of Obstetrics and Gynaecology* **102**: 282–7

Glazener CMA, Herbison GP, MacArthur C, et al (2006) New postnatal urinary incontinence: Obstetric and other risk factors in primiparae. *British Journal of Obstetrics and Gynaecology* **113**: 208–17

Gunn J, Lumley J, Chondros P, Young D (1998) Does an early postnatal check up improve maternal health? Results from a randomized controlled trial of Australian general practice. *British Journal of Obstetrics and Gynaecology* **105**: 991–7

Hager RM, Daltveit AK, Hofoss D, et al (2004) Complications of cesarean deliveries: Rates and risk factors. *American Journal of Obstetrics and Gynecology* **190**: 428–34

Hall Moran V, Edwards J, Dykes F, Downe S (2007) A systematic review of the nature of support for breast-feeding adolescent mothers. *Midwifery* **23**(2): 157–71

Hauck YL, Fenwick J, Dhaliwal SS, Butt J (2011) A Western Australian survey of breastfeeding initiation, prevalence and early cessation patterns. *Maternal and Child Health Journal* **15**(2): 260–8

Heslehurst N, Rankin J, Wilkinson JR, et al (2010) A nationally representative study of maternal obesity in England, UK: Trends in incidence and demographic inequalities in 619323 births, 1989–2007. *International Journal of Obesity* **34**: 420–8

Hoddinott P, Britten J, Pill R (2010) Why do interventions work in some places and not others: A breastfeeding support group trial. *Social Science and Medicine* **70**(5): 769–78

Hoddinott P, Pill R (1999) Qualitative study of decisions about infant feeding among women in east end of London. *British Medical Journal* **318**: 30–4

Hojberg KE, Salvig JD, Winlsow NA, Lose G, Secher NJ (1999) Urinary incontinence: Prevalence and risk factors at 16 weeks gestation. *British Journal of Obstetrics and Gynaecology* **106**: 842–50

Howie PW, Forsyth JS, Ogston SA, Clark A, du V Florey C (1990) Protective effect of breast feeding against infection. *British Medical Journal* **300**: 11–16

Information Centre (2011) I*nfant feeding Survey 2010. Early results*. Health and Social Care Information Centre, London

Joseph KS, Liu S, Rouleau J, Kirby RS, Kramer MS, Sauve R, Fraser WD, Young DC, Liston RM and the Maternal Health Study Group of the Canadian Perinatal Surveillance System (2010) Severe maternal morbidity in Canada, 2003 to 2007: Surveillance using routine hospitalization data and ICD-10CA codes. *Journal of Obstetrics and Gynaecology Canada* **32**(9): 837–46

Kayem G, Kurinczuk J, Lewis G, Golightly S, Brocklehurst P, Knight M (2011) Risk factors for progression from severe maternal morbidity to death: A national cohort study. *PLoS One* **6**(12): e29077

Kelly LS, Sheeder J, Stevens-Simon C (2005) Why lightning strikes twice: Postpartum resumption of sexual activity during adolescence. *Journal of Pediatric and Adolescent Gynecology* **18**: 327–35

Knight M, Kurinczuk JJ, Tufnell D, Brocklehurst P (2005) The UK Obstetric Surveillance System for rare disorders of pregnancy. *British Journal of Obstetrics and Gynaecology* **112**: 263–5

Lamont RF, Sobel JD, Kusanovic JP, Vaisbuch E, Mazaki-Tovi S, Kim SK, Uldbjerg N, Romero R (2011) Current debate on the use of antibiotic prophylaxis for caesarean section. *British Journal of Obstetrics and Gynaecology* **118**(2): 193–201

Larsson PG, Platz-Christensen JJ, Bergman B, et al (1991) Advantage or disadvantage of episiotomy compared with spontaneous perineal laceration. *Gynecologic and Obstetric Investigation* **31**: 213–6

Lewis G (ed) (2007) *The Confidential Enquiry into Maternal and Child Health (CEMACH). Saving mothers' lives: Reviewing maternal deaths to make motherhood safer 2003–2005. The Seventh Report on Confidential Enquiries into Maternal Deaths in the United Kingdom.* CEMACH, London

Lewis LN, Doherty DA, Hickey M, Skinner SR (2010) Predictors of sexual intercourse and rapid-repeat pregnancy among teenage mothers: An Australian prospective longitudinal study. *Medical Journal of Australia* **193**(6): 338–42

Lewis G, Drife J (eds) (2004) *Why mothers die 2000–2002. Sixth Report of the Confidential Enquiries into Maternal and Child Health.* Royal College of General Practitioners Press, London

Lopez LM, Hiller JE, Grimes DA (2010) Education for contraceptive use by women after childbirth. *CochraneDatabase of Systematic Reviews*, **1**: Art. No. CD001863

Luke B, Brown MB (2007) Elevated risks of pregnancy complications and adverse outcomes with increasing maternal age. *Human Reproduction* **22**(5): 1264– 72

MacArthur C, Glazener C, Wilson P, Herbison G, Gee H, et al (2001) Obstetric practice and faecal incontinence three months after delivery. *British Journal of Obstetrics and Gynaecology* **108**: 678–83

MacArthur C, Glazener CMA, Wilson PD, Lancashire RJ, Herbison GP, Grant AM (2006) Persistent urinary incontinence and delivery mode history: A six-year longitudinal study. *British Journal of Obstetrics and Gynaecology* **113**: 218–24

MacArthur C, Lewis G, Knox EG (1991) Health after childbirth. HMSO, London

MacArthur C, Lewis M, Knox EG, Crawford JS (1990) Epidural anaesthesia and long term backache after childbirth. *British Medical Journal* **301**: 9–12

MacArthur AJ, MacArthur C (2004) Incidence, severity and determinants of perineal pain after vaginal delivery: A prospective cohort study. *American Journal Obstetrics and Gynecology* **191**(4): 1199–204

MacArthur C, Winter H, Bick D, et al (2002) Effects of redesigned community postnatal care on women's health 4 months after birth: A cluster randomised controlled trial. *The Lancet* **359**: 378–85

MacArthur C, Winter HR, Bick DE et al (2003) Redesigning postnatal care; a randomised controlled trial of protocol based, midwifery led care focused on individual women's physical and psychological health needs. *Health Technology Assessment* **7**: No. 37

Marild S, Hansson S, Jodal U, et al (2004) Protective effect of breastfeeding against urinary tract infection. *Acta Paediatrica Scandinavica* **93**(2): 164–8

Milgrom J, Gemmill AW, Bilszta JL, et al (2008) Antenatal risk factors for postnatal depression: A large prospective study. *Journal of Affective Disorders* **108**(1–2): 147–57

Morrell C, Spiby H, Stewart P, Walters S, Morgan A (2000) Costs and effectiveness of community postnatal support workers: Randomized controlled trial. *British Medical Journal* **321**: 593–8

National Institute for Health and Clinical Excellence (2005) *Long acting reversible contraception: The effectiveness and appropriate use of long-acting reversible contraception. NICE clinical guideline 30.* National Collaborating Centre for Women's and Child Children's Health, London

National Institute for Health and Clinical Excellence (2006) *Routine postnatal care of women and their babies. NICE clinical guideline 37.* National Collaborating Centre for Primary Care, London

National Institute for Health and Clinical Excellence (2007) *Antenatal and postnatal mental health. NICE clinical guideline 45.* National Collaborating Centre for Mental Health, London

National Institute for Health and Clinical Excellence (2010a) *Pregnancy and complex social factors. NICE clinical guideline 110.* National Collaborating Centre for Women's and Children's Health, London

National Institute for Health and Clinical Excellence (2010b). *Weight management before, during and after pregnancy. Public Health guidance 27.* National Institute for Health and Clinical Excellence, London

Office for National Statistics (2011) *Infant and perinatal mortality in England and Wales by social and biological factors, 2010.* ONS, London

Paranjothy S, Broughton H, Adappa R, et al (2009) Teenage pregnancy: Who suffers? *Archives of Diseases of Childhood* **94**: 239

Phipps MG, Blume JD, DeMonner SM (2002) Young maternal age associated with increased risk of postneonatal death. *Obstetrics and Gynecology* **100**: 481

Rees JM, Lederman SA, Kiely JL (1996) Birth weight associated with lowest neonatal mortality: Infants of adolescent and adult mothers. *Pediatrics* **98**(6 Pt1): 1161

Reid M, Glazener C, Murray G, Taylor G (2002) A two centred pragmatic randomised controlled trial of two intervensions of postnatal support. *British Journal of Obstetrics and Gynaecology* **109**: 1164–70

Robertson E, Grace S, Wallington T, Stewart DE (2004) Antenatal risk factors for postpartum depression: A synthesis of recent literature. *General Hospital Psychiatry* **26**: 289–95

Sadashivaiah J, McLure H (2009) 18-G Tuohy needle can reduce the incidence of severe post-dural puncture headache. *Anaesthesia* **64**: 1379–80

Sadashivaiah J, Wilson R, McLure H, Lyons G (2010) Double-space combined spinal-epidural technique for elective caesarean section: A review of 10 years' experience in a UK teaching maternity unit. *International Journal of Obstetric Anesthesia* **19**(2):183–7

Sadauskaite-Kuehne V, Ludvigsson J, Padaiga Z, Jasinskiene E, Samuelsson U (2004) Longer breastfeeding is an independent protective factor against development of type 1 diabetes mellitus in childhood. *Diabetes Metabolism Research Review* **20**(2):150–7

Schutte JM, Steegers EA, Schuitemaker NW, et al (2010) Rise in maternal mortality in the Netherlands. *British Journal of Obstetrics and Gynaecology* **117**: 399–406

Shrim A, Ates S, Mallozzi A, et al (2011) Is young maternal age really a risk factor for adverse pregnancy outcome in a Canadian tertiary referral hospital? *Journal of Pediatric and Adolescent Gynecology* **24**(4): 218–22

Signorello LB, Harlow BL, Chekos AK, Repke JT (2001) Postpartum sexual functioning and its relationship to perineal trauma: A retrospective cohort study of primiparous women. *American Journal Obstetrics and Gynecology* **184**(5): 881–8

Social Exclusion Unit (1999) *Teenage pregnancy*. Social Exclusion Unit, London

Tucker CM, Wilson EK, Samandari G (2011). Infant feeding experiences among teen mothers in North Carolina: Findings from a mixed-methods study. *International Breastfeeding Journal* **6**: 14

Viktrup L, Rortveit G, Lose G (2006) Risk of stress urinary incontinence twelve years after the first pregnancy and delivery. *Obstetrics and Gynaecology* **108**: 248–54

Ward VP, Charlett A, Fagan J, Crawshaw SC (2008) Enhanced surgical site infection surveillance following caesarean section: Experience of a multicentre collaborative post-discharge system. *Journal of Hospital Infection* **70**(2): 166–73

World Health Organization (2006) *Pregnancy, childbirth, postpartum and newborn care: A guide for essential practice*. WHO Geneva

Chapter 6

Psychological and social issues

Introduction

This chapter outlines the short and long-term social and psychological outcomes for teenage mothers and mothers of advanced maternal age in terms of their own wellbeing, that of their baby and their wider social context. There are many factors that determine any woman's decision about the timing of motherhood, ranging from individual reasons (e.g. readiness, health issues, biological pressures, etc.) to familial factors (e.g. stable relationship with partner, partner's readiness, financial stability, etc.), and societal influences (such as social acceptability, support, etc.) (Benzies et al, 2006). Being ready to share a baby and start a family does not necessarily have to be related to age, because it is influenced by personal choice, beliefs and values.

Section 1
Teenage pregnancy: Long-term outcomes and parenting

Anja Wittkowski and Aleksandra Staneva

Introduction

For a typical teenager, adolescence is a time for much physical, emotional, cognitive and psychological development, along with an increased move towards a more independent life. Becoming pregnant at this stage in life significantly alters an adolescent girl's developmental pathway (e.g. Flanagan et al, 1995). Although all expectant women will have to adjust to the new role of becoming a mother, some adolescent or teenage mothers-to-be may not be as well prepared for pregnancy and motherhood as women in the later stages of their reproductive lives. For example, during pregnancy, some teenage girls may engage in risky health behaviours, such as drinking and smoking, eat less well, and engage less with appropriate prenatal care (Mayers and Siegler, 2004). They may also live in inadequate conditions and receive little support from the baby's father or from their own family (Mayers and Siegler, 2004). When these factors impinge on teenage girls who are pregnant or who have just given birth, the mental health and wellbeing of both the mother and infant can be at risk of having a poorer short and long-term psychological outcome. However, the context of the pregnancy also determines behaviour. Whether or not the pregnancy was planned, or indeed wanted, may influence the woman's decision to look after her own health and that of her growing fetus. Studies suggest that an unplanned pregnancy can be experienced as a traumatic event by a young woman who may decide against a termination if this is unacceptable to her, her family and her wider social group (e.g. Faber, 1991).

Not all teenage girls show risky antenatal or postnatal health behaviours or experience adverse social circumstances. However, irrespective of whether or not their pregnancy was planned or wanted, societal views of adolescent pregnancy and motherhood are largely characterised by beliefs of there being a perceived negative impact on the mother, the baby and ultimately wider society (Wiemann et al, 2005). For example, teenage mothers are often seen by society as continuing a certain cycle of disadvantage: they come from a disadvantaged background and their children will grow up in similar circumstances, which then makes them vulnerable to also having children early. This 'cycle of disadvantage' is not just a media phenomenon; it is a reality for some teenage mothers who may become pregnant earlier than planned as a result of pre-existing psychosocial problems, poor decision making and family dysfunction (e.g. Breheny and Stephens, 2008; Harden et al, 2009). Given the relatively high teenage pregnancy rate in the UK and the USA, there has been much debate about teenage pregnancy being a social problem that requires early intervention (e.g. Mayers and Siegler, 2004).

This view of teenage childbearing perpetuating psychosocial problems is supported by the relationship between teenage pregnancy and poor parenting competence (Flanagan et al, 1995), poor psychological functioning (Sommer et al, 1993), low socioeconomic status, unemployment, low levels of educational attainment (Coley and Chase-Lansdale, 1998), and in some cases, child neglect and abuse (Garrett and Tidwell, 1999). Furthermore, the media have helped to increase this notion of perceived and actual stigma experienced by adolescent mothers, which may result in them being at an increased risk of social isolation (Wiemann et al, 2005). For example, teenage mothers reported that they felt discriminated against by healthcare professionals, other people, and socially (Kelly, 1996). Judgemental views about teenage girls making wrong decisions (with regard to becoming pregnant or continuing with a pregnancy) and coming from the 'wrong' family are still dominant beliefs in our society. The idea that society is wrong in condemning and stigmatising teenage mothers is far less prevalent, but has been voiced (Kelly, 1996).

Parenting behaviours shown by teenage mothers

The concept of a cycle of disadvantage is based on the assumption that teenage motherhood is both a predictor and an outcome of 'social exclusion' (Breheny and Stephens, 2008). Whilst this may not be true for all teenage mothers, research findings indicate that for some teenage mothers this disadvantage is represented under a 'triple jeopardy', i.e. when low parenting confidence, together with high parenting stress, is underpinned by inappropriate expectations towards parenting (East et al, 1994). For example, being young when giving birth to a baby has been linked to particular parenting behaviours, which are characterised by being less accepting of the child, being angrier with the growing child (aged between 12 and 50 months) and using more punitive child-control strategies (Crockenberg, 1987). In general, studies have noted that the children of teenage mothers appeared to be at increased risk of subsequent adverse outcomes from infancy to adolescence, potentially due to their mothers being less aware of normal developmental milestones in their babies and infants (Letourneau et al, 2004). This lack of awareness may be linked to disinterest, poorer utilisation of health visiting and other healthcare professional support, a poorer exchange of guidance amongst teenage mothers as well as perceived stigma, all of which reduce the chances of the mother seeking appropriate and timely advice (Crockenberg, 1986).

A study examining key parenting behaviours amongst 1702 low income North American mothers observed that teenage mothers were significantly less supportive, more detached, more intrusive, and more hostile with their infants than older mothers (over 19 years), irrespective of ethnicity/race, educational attainment, family type, income, and the child's sex (Berlin et al, 2002). It is possible that the many demands of their own developmental transitions to adulthood and its responsibilities, do not allow teenage mothers sufficient resources to attend sensitively to their children's needs (Berlin et al, 2002).

Adolescent mothers have been found to vocalise less with their infants, to be less flexible, to be more likely to give inappropriate stimulation and to be more likely to mistreat or neglect their child (Brooks-Gunn and Furstenberg, 1986; Crockenberg, 1986; East and Felice, 1990; Osofsky et al, 1993). It is widely recognised that a mother's ability to read accurately and respond to her baby's cues is paramount to the infant's cognitive, social and emotional development (Belsky, 1999). Whilst not all studies suggest that teenage mothers are insensitive or unresponsive towards their infants, they do not seem to be as good at cue-recognition as older mothers (Berlin et al, 2002). One of the reasons for poorer interactions with their babies could be the teenage mother's lack of appropriate role models, possibly because their own mothers or grandmothers did not provide them with appropriate models of mothering. However, teenage mothers, on account of their age, may also lack the cognitive or emotional maturity necessary for consistent, contingent responsiveness to their infant's normal demands, which involves prioritising the infant's needs above your own (Osofsky et al, 1993; East et al, 1994). Sommer and colleagues (1993) described this process as 'cognitive readiness' for parenting, which combines an adequate knowledge of child development with a positive attitude to becoming a parent and a good enough understanding of appropriate parenting practices. Whilst the degree of cognitive readiness may not be solely age-dependent, an adolescent girl's ability to parent well may be strongly influenced by certain risk factors that are associated with her young age, namely higher economic dependency on her own family or the welfare state, including the possible lack of social support from her family or the baby's father.

Risk factors for becoming a mother as a teenager

Researchers have tried to identify some of the factors that increase the likelihood of teenage girls becoming pregnant, sometimes deliberately. In their systematic review, Harden and colleagues (2009) discovered three main themes that were linked to early parenthood:

- Dislike of school (because of academic demands, being bullied, or difficulties in following the rules and regulations of the school institution).
- Poor economic and material circumstances.
- An unhappy childhood characterised by family breakdown, divorce, and violence, as well as the teenager's own lack of confidence, low self-esteem, high anxiety levels and low expectations for the future (in terms of getting an education, getting a job).

Having a baby may therefore be viewed as one solution to escape unhappy circumstances. Other risk factors identified in the literature include coming from a poor, dysfunctional or single parent family, living in unstable or inadequate arrangements, and living in a violent household or neighbourhood (Letourneau et al, 2007). Living in lower socioeconomic circumstances in disadvantaged neighbourhoods increased the likelihood of teenage girls getting pregnant, but this may in part be related to growing up in single parent households and to their own mother having been a teenager when giving birth to them. Miller and colleagues (2001) also identified that being the victim of physical and sexual abuse was linked to teenage pregnancy. These socioeconomic factors not only increase the risk of becoming pregnant, but also point towards the continuation of the cycle of disadvantage. Whilst most mothers-to-be have to adapt to their given socioeconomic situation, there is one important factor that can influence their own wellbeing and that of their infant, namely, the family context. In her study using observations of children born to sisters (who were either teenagers or not when they got pregnant), Turley (2003) concluded that the disadvantages associated with having been born to a younger mother are not due to the mother's age at the birth of the baby, but rather to her disadvantaged family background (including educational attainment, income, number of children in the household, and marital status, especially divorce).

The family context in which children grow up influences their ability to form good and appropriate attachments or relationships with other people, which in turn will enhance or hinder their ability to develop psychologically and learn to cope with stressful life events. Naturally, not all teenage mothers will come from disadvantaged backgrounds or remain disadvantaged after the birth of their baby. Despite some difficult socioeconomic conditions, some adolescent mothers do well enough as mothers. The protective factors that appear to increase psychological resilience in adolescent mothers include being able to draw on strong social support (from their own family, grandparents, their partner and his family, etc.), being able to continue education, having a stable relationship with the baby's father, having high self-esteem and good problem-solving skills, alongside an infant with an 'easy' temperament (Osofsky et al, 1993). Montgomery (2001) also noted that financial stability, a stable relationship and an ability to hold down a job determined the readiness to become mothers in adolescents who planned their pregnancies. These advantageous psychological and practical resources may allow a teenage mother to adapt more successfully to being a mother and to manage the many, sometimes stressful, challenges of early parenthood.

The impact of mood on teenage mothers and their parenting behaviours and attachment

In their review of postnatal depression (PND) in adolescent mothers, Reid and Meadows-Oliver (2007) revealed that over 53% of teenage mothers experienced PND, which is considerably higher than the generally accepted prevalence of 13%. In their review of 12 studies, teenage mothers who perceived themselves as being more stressed were more likely to report increased levels of PND. More family conflict, fewer social support networks, and low self-esteem were also associated with increased rates of depressive symptoms in these younger mothers. In addition, these mothers were more likely to report not feeling confident as a parent or gratified with being a mother. The lower their mood the less they appeared to interact positively with their infants, which in turn contributed to a host of physical, emotional and behavioural problems in the child's later life (East and Felice, 1990; Leadbeater et al, 1996; Schmidt et al, 2005; Cox et al, 2008).

In a prospective study of 625 adolescent mothers who were followed up four years after delivery (Schmidt et al, 2005), the prevalence of moderate to severe depressive symptoms was highest at three months after the birth and then steadily declined over time, which is comparable to that noted in all new mothers (e.g. Kumar and Robson, 1984; Cooper and Murray, 1998). However, it has been widely suggested that teenage mothers display more instances of depression than mothers in general (e.g. Osofsky et al, 1993) and the higher than usual prevalence rate described above supports this assumption. Schmidt and colleagues (2005) reported a PND prevalence rate of 57% in their sample of mothers. It is therefore advisable that healthcare providers ask teenage mothers about their mood in the postpartum period and ideally continue to enquire about their feelings until the baby is at least 6 months old. Regular meetings between teenage mothers and their named health visitor could facilitate the development of a trusting relationship, which would allow these young mothers openly to discuss their feelings following the birth of their baby. Through regular reviews, the health visitor can assist these mothers to monitor their own mood and to identify possible triggers to, as well as factors that help to maintain, low mood. Mood diaries can help the teenage mother to identify patterns and variability in her mood. There are various self-help guides available on the internet (e.g. www.cci.health.wa.gov.au; www.getselfhelp.co.uk) that can be used by these mothers on their own or in conjunction with health visitor appointments.

The ability to relate well to others not only fosters the bond between people, including mother and baby, but also contributes to the ability to elicit appropriate care giving. A strong vulnerability factor for the development of ante and postnatal depression in the transition to parenthood (Figueiredo et al, 2006) is the attachment style the mother adopts. One study observed that, compared to older mothers, pregnant teenagers were significantly more likely to have an insecure attachment style characterised by enmeshed, angry/dismissive or fearful relationship behaviours (Figueiredo et al, 2006). Furthermore, perceived closeness with significant others has also been linked to the developing attachment between the adolescent mother-to-be and her unborn baby. Better attachments with the developing fetus appear to be positively influenced by being married, having more contact with the baby's father and having a close relationship with their own mothers, all of which means the mother may develop a good bond with her baby (Wayland and Tate, 1993). Consequently, it is reasonable to assume that activities encouraging the pregnant woman to focus her attention on the developing fetus may enhance attachment (Grace, 1989; Figueiredo et al, 2006).

Given the fact that teenage mothers have to adjust to their own ongoing developmental issues whilst adjusting to motherhood, they may indeed find themselves at greater risk of developing PND. When considering this possibility, the teenage mother's social and socioeconomic background is likely to influence her ability to cope, which is why it is important to screen for antenatal and postnatal depression in younger mothers (Schmidt et al, 2005). Mother-centred interventions have been shown to promote successful adaptation for adolescent mothers and their children. Comprehensive, multidisciplinary care addressing the psychosocial, medical, developmental and educational needs of adolescent mothers and their children appears to facilitate positive outcomes (Letourneau et al, 2004).

Long-term outcomes for infants of teenage mothers

Many studies have explored the long-term effects on the children of adolescent mothers. A general finding is that maternal age has an indirect effect on the child's cognitive and language abilities, in particular expressive language and language comprehension (Brooks-Gunn and Chase-Lansdale, 1995; Keown et al, 2001). This observation can in part be explained by some of the above-mentioned parenting and interaction behaviours (e.g. Rafferty et al, 2011). For example, in a study with low income younger mothers it was found that they were less supportive during play with their 14-month-old toddlers compared to mothers aged 20 or older. In their examination of the physical, academic and psychological outcomes for children of adolescent mothers, Brooks-Gunn and Furstenberg (1986) found that intellectual differences in children born to teenage mothers became more pronounced as their children developed and were particularly evident in behavioural differences (including problems with activity levels, hostility and other challenging behaviours). Similarly, in a Canadian study (Letourneau et al, 2004), which examined longitudinal data on over 2300 children born to either adolescent or older mothers, levels of anxiety and hyperactivity were found to be higher for the children of teenage mothers. Compared to older, more educated mothers, adolescent mothers displayed less than optimal parenting interactions, higher levels of depression and their children were more likely to experience developmental challenges (Letourneau et al, 2007). However, adolescent mothers who were able to use consistent and more positive parenting techniques were observed to have considerably less anxious and less hyperactive children. It is of course feasible that the increased stress, time demands, and daily hassles associated with attending school while taking care of small children negatively impact on the teenage mother's ability to parent her child consistently and effectively (Letourneau et al, 2007).

Furthermore, an Australian prospective study of over 5000 mother–child dyads identified that the 14-year-old offspring of mothers who were aged 18 and younger at the time of birth, were more likely to show disturbed psychological behaviours and poorer school performances including a poorer reading ability. These 14-year-olds were also more likely to engage in crime and adverse health behaviours, such as regular smoking and drinking (Shaw et al, 2005). These associations between young maternal age at birth and the outcomes for their own teenage children were largely explained by various socioeconomic factors (maternal education, family income, and living conditions, including the neighbourhood the family lived in), family structure (living with own parents or extended family), marital status, maternal health, health practices and depression (Shaw et al, 2005). This study appears to support the notion of teenage mothers continuing the cycle of disadvantage. Although the long-term outcomes of infants born to teenage mothers may not appear favourable given these studies, they are not necessarily always negative. The teenage mother's own psychological resilience and family system can help her to become an engaging, consistent parent. Health professionals can also contribute to ensure that the developmental pathway for children of teenage mothers is a good one by engaging these mothers in appropriate antenatal and postnatal care with a focus on the mother–infant bond and interaction.

Transition to and experience of motherhood in teenagers

Whilst all expectant women have to make the transition to a new role and to adjust psychologically to becoming and then being a mother, the experience of motherhood may be perceived as more challenging by adolescent girls. The appropriate adjustment to motherhood will certainly depend on the social context the new mother finds herself in. Family and partner support, financial stability (possibly offered by her family, her partner or his family), appropriate living conditions for her and her baby, and the availability of childcare (especially if she continues her education) are important factors that facilitate appropriate adjustment in mothers of any age. However, adjustment to motherhood is also influenced by a range of psychological factors, including maternal expectations and general resilience (Breen and McLean, 2010).

In a meta-synthesis of 12 qualitative studies focusing on adolescent mothers' experiences, Clemmens (2003) identified five general themes. The reality of motherhood was, perhaps realistically, viewed as 'bringing hardship'; adolescent mothers thought that motherhood would be easier than it actually was and many teenagers viewed it as a responsibility from which they could not get away. They also expressed feeling stuck and tied down, feelings that have also been reported by non-teenage mothers (Clemmens, 2003). However, adolescent mothers also verbalised the experience of feeling torn apart between being an adolescent and a mother, which has been described as 'living in two worlds'. Most teenage mothers expressed this conflict as resulting in feelings of anxiety, alienation and isolation. The conflict between being your own person and a person who has to consistently prioritise an infant's needs above your own (for a considerable amount of time given the baby's initial dependence) has been widely reported in the literature (Nicolson, 1999). In the case of teenage mothers, the very fact that they are still adolescents, with a less defined sense of self, may be crucial here. Their own emotional and cognitive immaturity influences their ability to negotiate this internal conflict between roles. They may still be in a developmental stage in their life cycle during which they are used to prioritising and fulfilling their own needs ahead of others. On the other hand, a significant number of adolescent mothers in this meta-synthesis described themselves as changing and growing through the experience of being a mother, stating that they have found a 'voice in learning to speak up for what they believed in' and thinking of their lives differently (Clemmens, 2003). This experience was considered as providing them with an identity that 'has been lost' as well as improving the relationship between adolescent mothers and their families (Arensen, 1994).

A crucial factor in an adolescent's ability to cope with motherhood was the importance of social support, with many studies highlighting the positive influence of social support provided by community programmes (Clemmens, 2003). Partner and family support can also play a valuable role, if it is available. In addition, community programmes, as well as significant others, can provide the mother with additional opportunities to learn how to interact well with her baby and establish a strong, reciprocal bond (Brophy-Herb and Honig, 1999).

As the adjustment to motherhood can be challenging, even under optimal psychosocial circumstances, it is important to recognise the role that prenatal and postnatal perceptions of stress can play in maternal adjustment. While the relationship between perinatal stress and maternal adjustment has been explored among adult mothers, few studies have examined the effects of stress on adolescent mothers. For new mothers, stress is a common response to increasing demands and challenging transformations. However, increased stress affects the quality and experiences of pregnancy and parenting as well as maternal and child outcomes (Holub et al, 2007). In a longitudinal project involving 154 teenage mothers, interviewed during their pregnancy and four months after birth, Holub and colleagues (2007) identified that those adolescent mothers who experienced high perinatal stress as well as high parenting stress, also showed lower maternal adjustment, less positive feelings about motherhood, less infant care, and lower parenting competence. All of these observations have adverse effects on both maternal and child outcomes, including the mother–infant bond. These findings support the need for appropriate psychological interventions offered to teenage mothers vulnerable to environmental stress and emotional distress.

Interestingly, another longitudinal study investigating the relationship between teenage childbearing and overall psychological distress found that the experience of adolescent mothers did not appear to cause high levels of stress *per se*, particularly postnatally. It seemed that some teenage mothers were highly distressed prior to becoming pregnant compared to their peers and they continued to experience distress after birth and into early and middle adulthood. An important observation in this study was that distress *per se* during adolescence did not increase the likelihood of those teenagers becoming pregnant, except among economically disadvantaged teens (Mollborn and Morningstar, 2009). It could be argued that the degree of distress they experienced made them engage in riskier behaviours that resulted in the pregnancy, or that they viewed the idea of having a baby as a way to escape their distressing situation. This finding, opposite to generally held beliefs, confirms that it is not the age, but the family psychosocial and socioeconomic context that influences a teenager's decision to become a mother, and her subsequent parenting.

The importance of support

Social support is crucial for all mothers in their efforts to adjust to a new role as primary caregiver to a baby. Support by their partner, in particular, and by their wider family in general is important not only during the initial weeks following the birth of the baby, but also in terms of ongoing parenting. In addition, familial support may be particularly critical for providing both emotional and practical assistance to the teenage mother, at least initially until her parenting confidence and self-reliance grow (Nath et al, 1991). However, teenage mothers appear to prefer informal support offered by friends and family over formal support, which may explain their reluctance to engage with health visiting services (Crockenberg, 1986). This reluctance to engage with services may also be influenced by perceptions of being stigmatised either by the media, society as a whole or by healthcare professionals in particular, as outlined earlier.

Adolescent fathers are typically two to three years older than the mothers (Beers and Hollo, 2009). Although there are many negative stereotypes surrounding adolescent fathers, studies suggest that most fathers want to be involved with their infants, which positively impacts on both parents' ability to meet the needs of the child effectively (Wayland and Tate, 1993; Letourneau et al, 2004). Adolescent mothers rated their child's father as the second most valuable source of support, after their own mother (Beers and Hollo, 2009). In addition, adolescent mothers who have a good, communicative and flexible relationship with their own mothers tend to exhibit more positive parenting behaviours and lower levels of depression. This appears to be influenced by emotional, economic and practical support, opportunities for modelling parenting skills and also educational support (Beers and Hollo, 2009). Being able to draw on family and partner for support in raising a child is clearly important for a mother's wellbeing, and that of her developing baby. For example, partner support has been associated with greater responsiveness to infants and greater maternal satisfaction with life (Unger and Wandersman, 1988), possibly because it enhances the adjustment to parenting and the quality of the adolescent mother–infant relationship (Samuels et al, 1994). Additionally, grandparents play a unique and important role in the lives of teenage parents (Samuels et al, 1994). This supportive relationship appears to reduce stress among adolescent mothers, and it also enhances the mother–infant relationship, which in turn promotes infant development (Osofsky et al, 1993).

Various studies demonstrate that social support acts as a protective factor for the teenage mother. For example, higher levels of social support have been linked to better coping, better parenting and lower depressive symptoms, which then positively influence a mother's sense of competence. Higher levels of support are naturally linked to feeling less isolated and possibly less stigmatised (Wiemann et al, 2005). All of these factors have been linked to better developmental outcomes for the child, which has been evidenced in general improvements in emotional tone and wellbeing (Mayers et al, 2008) as well as more prosocial behaviours in infants (Ensor and Hughes, 2010). Hence, it can be assumed that the availability and subsequent use of social support may serve as protection from the potential adverse effects of teenage parenting. A supportive person may act as a buffer, alleviating the psychological, financial and emotional impact on the mother, while also providing an indirect source of support for the child (Letourneau et al, 2004).

A review of the research on the support needs of adolescent mothers and the sources available to them revealed that teenage mothers and their children are often exposed to a whole range of psychological, social and economic difficulties, such as poverty, residential instability, violent and crime-ridden communities and less social support than adult mothers (Letourneau et al, 2004). Typical sources of support for adolescents were primarily informal networks, such as family, partner and friends, and to a lesser extent, professionals. In general, adolescents' perceptions of family support were often positively associated with maternal behaviour, and life and parental satisfaction. This suggests that adolescent mothers may be more responsive to the effects of social support than older mothers, and their satisfaction may be a good predictor of maternal competence (Letourneau et al, 2004). Many adolescent mothers indicated that their needs for support should be addressed through professional support and education, such as building knowledge about child health, development and behaviour; parental skills; confidence and psychological wellbeing; contraception; relationships; and employability. Adolescent girls need to be supported in their transition to parenthood, and special care should be provided for mothers who are socially isolated (Aujoulat et al, 2010).

Interventions

A systematic review of controlled trials and qualitative studies in the UK on teenage pregnancy and social disadvantage, examined the impact of interventions on teenage pregnancy (Harden et al, 2009). By addressing the disadvantage associated with early parenthood, this review suggests that early childhood interventions and youth programmes can help to reduce unintended teenage pregnancy. For example, the risk of teenage pregnancy was lower among individuals receiving an intervention, compared to standard practice. However, intervention programmes not only focus on reducing teenage pregnancy in the first place, but also on improving the possible outcomes for the teenage mother and her child. These programmes focus either on the social setting of the teenage mother, such as the home, school or wider community (Leoturneoau et al, 2004) or they specifically target the mother or the infant considered at risk (Deutscher et al, 2006).

A number of intervention studies illustrate that teenage mothers can successfully improve their interactions with their infants and thereby place them on a better developmental trajectory. In a home visiting community-based programme, which involved 84 US adolescents aged 12 to 18 years, the intervention programme improved mothers' parenting attitudes and school continuation (Barnet et al, 2007). Another teenage parent–infant programme targeting low-income, high-risk teenage mothers confirmed that mothers who received the intervention interacted better with their infants by being more responsive, more emotionally available and more directive in their interactions. In addition, infants were found to be much more interested in interacting with their mothers, responded more positively to physical contact and bonded better with their caregivers (Mayers et al, 2008). The findings remained true even for mothers who were quite depressed, confirming that it is possible to improve mother–infant interaction without directly addressing maternal depression. Similarly, in another project aimed at enhancing the interactions of teenage mothers and their at-risk children, mothers who received the interventions, such as a relationship-focused curriculum offered in 24 sessions, showed a significant improvement in responsiveness, less directiveness and were more facilitative of child language development, confirming the effectiveness of maternal-focused interventions to influence child outcome (Deutscher et al, 2006).

Whilst the evidence suggests that interventions can be beneficial to teenage mothers and their infants despite possible socioeconomic or psychological disadvantages, there are some important factors to be considered when working with this group of mothers. Carter and colleagues (1991) warn that interventions with teenage mothers may present a range of challenges, such as teenagers refusing advice or instructions as a result of pressing struggles for independence. Additionally, teenagers may be faced with the added issue of responding to other people's needs, as they are concerned primarily with caring for themselves in line with their own developmental stage in the life cycle.

Brophy-Herb and Honig (1999) advocate a focus on maternal reflexivity (the mother's ability to reflect on herself and her child), by permitting young mothers to realise that they can be in charge of their own decisions on how to parent their children, which can be similar or different to their own upbringing. In their controlled study, 27 teenage mothers participated in a three month intervention of home visits to enhance maternal skills and sensitivity. Findings suggested that most adolescent mothers had difficulty in being reflective, but the ones who benefited from the intervention scored higher on cognitive growth and language-fostering behaviours, as well as feeding and play interactions with their infants.

It is important to note that qualitative studies revealed that teenagers themselves desired close personal relationships with mentors and programme staff, practical support with child care and housing, and health and parenting education (Cox et al, 2005). The most successful interventions, despite some design limitations, usually follow best practice components such as providing comprehensive, multidisciplinary care, as well as addressing the psychological, medical, developmental and educational needs of adolescent mothers, their children and the extended family (Beers and Hollo, 2009). If adequately supported, a teenage pregnancy does not have to be at risk, adding to the evidence of the role that provision and mediation of support play in promoting wellbeing, particularly in adolescent mothers. Therefore, interventions that build upon strengths, and promote personal and familial wellbeing can have a positive influence on teenage parenting (Dunst et al, 1986). Factors associated with a better adjustment to parenting during the teenage years are summarised in *Box 6.1*.

Box 6.1. Factors affecting teenage pregnancy and parenthood

- Context of pregnancy, including cultural practices, etc.
- Support (baby's father and his family, own family, peers, wider support system at school or in the community, etc.)
- Living arrangements whilst pregnant and once baby is born
- Plans for continuing education
- Expectations for future, career, etc.
- Current and past mood and psychological resilience, including coping with life events and nature of life events (victim of abuse, crime or bullying, etc.)
- Knowledge of parenting and caring for a baby, including the presence of attachment or parenting figures in mother's life

Very young mothers

- Current support systems, types of support (emotional, financial, practical, etc.) and frequency mother can access these systems
- Living arrangements
- Financial support
- Relationship with infant including the way mother and infant interact with each other
- Knowledge of parenting skills and confidence and competence in parenting

Conclusion

The literature on teenage pregnancy and motherhood is quite extensive, with many studies originating in the US. Given that the US has the highest prevalence rate of teenage pregnancies in the world, it is not surprising that so much research originates there. The extent of the literature may also be a reflection of the ongoing debate about teenage pregnancies and motherhood being a problem for society because of the perceived disadvantages to the infant's developmental chances, which may contribute to the cycle of disadvantage outlined earlier. In this section, the focus was on the psychological and social impact of teenage pregnancy on the child once born, rather than on the growing literature surrounding the impact of maternal stress on the developing fetus. Since most interventions are aimed at preventing teenage pregnancies or improving their outcomes by focusing on the mother–infant interaction and general relationship, this focus was appropriate.

As outlined in this section, the impact of teenage pregnancy and motherhood should be taken seriously, but the teenage mother should not be blamed or condemned for her choices. Instead she should be seen in the social context in which she presents and with the psychological strengths or weaknesses that she brings on her journey to motherhood. Health professionals need to be creative in engaging these sometimes very vulnerable young women so that they can benefit from a range of interventions that teach them appropriate parenting and interaction skills and increase their confidence, as well as competence, as mothers.

Discussion questions

- What is meant by the 'cycle of disadvantage' in relation to teenage mothers?
- What type of parenting behaviours do teenage mothers tend to show?
- What risk factors increase the likelihood of a teenage girl becoming a mother?
- What impact does mood have on teenage mothers' parenting behaviours?
- What are the long-term outcomes for the infants of teenage mothers?
- What helps and what hinders the transition to motherhood in teenage mothers?
- Why is postnatal support important?

Section 2
Advanced maternal age

Anja Wittkowski and Aleksandra Staneva

Introduction

Within the literature, it is relatively clear what is meant by teenage pregnancy, but the same cannot be said about advanced maternal age. Older women are considered to be an at risk group in terms of both maternal and neonatal outcomes because an increased maternal age carries with it an increased obstetric risk. However, studies are inconsistent in terms of defining older mothers, with some studies considering women over 30 years of age as older and others using 35 as a cut-off point for advance maternal age (e.g. Dobrzykowski and Stern, 2003; Carolan and Nelson, 2007). While authors have suggested differentiating between first-time mothers above 35, above 40 and above 45, most researchers simply include older mothers in their studies unless they specifically target this age group. This means that the older mother is often hidden in studies on motherhood because she will just be one in a range of mothers of different ages asked to share their views. In contrast to the quite extensive literature on teenage mothers, it seems that far less is known about the psychological adjustment of older mothers and most of the studies reported here are based on interviews of small groups of women. Therefore, this is an area that requires further exploration to help us fully understand the psychological and social impact of motherhood on women, their children, their families and wider society.

There are many reasons why some women become mothers at a later stage in their reproductive life cycle. For some, delayed motherhood may be an informed choice. Meisenhelder and Meservey (1987) examined reasons for delaying childbirth in women aged 29 to 38 years who completed a range of measures 3–11 months postnatally. They identified that needing time to develop oneself, a career, or marriage were factors in the women's decision-making process alongside infertility problems or only having met or married their partner recently. Late or second marriages following divorce may provide the psychological and socioeconomic stability that enable a woman to pursue motherhood at an advanced age (Benzies et al, 2006). Economic factors clearly influence these women's decisions regarding motherhood, with career advancement and the desire for financial stability often being cited as reasons for their delay (Berryman and Windridge, 1991a). In stark contrast to adolescent mothers, this group of women appears to decide when they want to become mothers; they plan and prepare financially as well as psychologically. Older mothers do not appear to present with the same psychological or social risk factors, including poverty, instability and family dysfunction.

While a woman's desire to provide a psychologically stable and financially secure home environment for her pregnant self and her developing child is very sensible, pregnancy at an advanced age is not always welcomed by UK society. Various studies have examined the social discourses relating to older mothers and, comparable to teenage mothers, the prevailing attitudes appear to be negative (e.g. Hadfield et al, 2007). For example, Shaw and Giles (2009) studied narratives used in the UK media over a one-week period in 2006 and noted a general disapproval of delayed motherhood: older mothers were portrayed as an 'indulgent generation' that deliberately put 'motherhood on ice'. Older mothers are also often perceived by the media and possibly wider society as 'unnatural'. Although this view may in part be explained by the media's reporting of the use of assisted reproductive technology by women of extreme advanced maternal age (postmenopause), as in the case of a 60-year-old mother of twins (Campbell, 2011), it seems that overall the advantages of being a mother above the age of 35 are not discussed or indeed celebrated in the media (Hadfield et al, 2007).

Although there are established medical risks associated with advanced maternal age, there are also a number of advantages. Older mothers are often more highly educated and enjoy a higher socioeconomic status compared to younger women. They often are in good physical health (in preparation for pregnancy), engage in appropriate health behaviours during pregnancy, seek prenatal care early and engage with antenatal and postnatal care providers (Viau, 2002). In contrast with teenage mothers, older women display a greater degree of psychological readiness for motherhood. Older mothers tend to express positive attitudes about pregnancy and motherhood. Life-span developmental theory (Smith and Bates, 1999) suggests that adults in their 30s have managed to shift the focus from their family of origin to their own home environment, by settling down with a partner. By successfully separating from their family of origin, they are more likely to develop the psychological readiness to start their own family. Their maturity, independence and life experience influence their parenting orientations and abilities as well as their psychological resilience to cope with the challenges of parenthood. Planning for a pregnancy, wanting to become pregnant and wanting to become a mother are important factors distinguishing this group of mothers from teenage mothers. Teenage girls may not embark on motherhood with the same degree of readiness, or practical and psychological resources.

Although women of advanced maternal age may be prepared to become mothers psychologically and socially, they may be less aware of age-related risk factors. Carolan and Nelson (2007) interviewed 22 first-time mothers, aged 35 and over, at three time points (35–38 weeks of gestation, 10–14 days postpartum, and 6–8 months postpartum) and noted that women realised they were at risk, hoped for reassurance, dealt with uncertainty and eventually got through it. Research clearly indicates that the successful adjustment to parenthood is related to women negotiating these risks. According to Lampinen and colleagues (2009), being 'at risk' is a label given to women of advanced maternal age because of pregnancy-related medical risk factors, which can make these women feel quite anxious during pregnancy. However, this concern may be eased by their desire to be as well informed as possible; hence, they are often seen to be avid information gatherers and proactive healthcare seekers (Viau, 2002). It seems obvious that the way information is shared by healthcare providers, and the attitudes they hold about older mothers, contribute to women's ability to cope with their concerns and anxieties about their own wellbeing and that of their fetus, and their adjustment after birth. Although the fear of losing a baby has to be managed by all mothers-to-be, the risks of medical complications are greater in this age group.

Short and long-term outcomes for infants of older mothers

Some older women (and men) may have to overcome fertility problems in order to become parents. In some cases, particularly among postmenopausal women, the use of reproductive technological advances in older mothers is highly controversial (e.g. Campbell, 2011). However, evidence suggests that in terms of parenting behaviours, older mothers may display superior skills compared with their younger counterparts. Appropriate parenting behaviours are of course linked to better short- and long-term outcomes for the developing child.

In contrast to teenage mothers, older mothers appear to have psychosocial advantages, possibly because often they are better informed and educated, and are wealthier (e.g. McMahon et al, 2011). Since older mothers may be concerned about their own and their fetus's wellbeing (e.g. Viau, 2002), they engage in various health-promoting behaviours and independently initiate adaptive changes and thereby promote a healthy pregnancy. This already places the child on a better developmental pathway. Older mothers may perceive the demands of looking after a baby as more tiring but they also express more pleasure in their parenting role compared to younger mothers, irrespective of their baby having been born prematurely or at full term (Ragozin et al, 1982).

In addition, older mothers have been identified as providing better nurturing environments and interactions for their developing infants, which positively impact on their development and translate into better educational and behavioural outcomes. In their longitudinal study of 1025 children, Fergusson and Woodward (1999) assessed the influence of maternal age on the educational and psychosocial outcomes of children once they turned 18 years of age. Increasing maternal age was linked to significant reductions in risks of educational under-achievement, juvenile crime, substance misuse, and mental health problems. This study stressed that although maternal age was an important influence on the psychosocial adjustment of these young adults, other factors also contributed. Not only do older mothers appear to be more nurturing and supportive and ensure more stable home environments, they also seem to have more confidence in their parenting abilities and hence use more effective and more positive child-rearing practices.

We can therefore conclude that, whilst advanced maternal age appears to contribute indirectly to better child outcomes, age *per se* does not lead to women being better mothers. Many other psychosocial factors play important roles in the adjustment to motherhood, such as whether the pregnancy was planned and desired, and whether delaying childbearing was voluntary. Harker and Thorpe (1992) stress that the context is crucial; a pregnancy may follow recurrent miscarriage or be conceived through *in vitro* fertilisation. Healthcare providers should therefore pay attention to a wide range of factors, such as a woman's education, financial situation, the quality of her (marital) relationship with the baby's father, her overall social status and home environment as well as the availability of a social network.

Impact of mood on older mothers and their parenting behaviours and attachment

As outlined above, older mothers appear to show relatively positive interactions and parenting behaviours towards their infants and developing children, often in the context of predictable, stable, nurturing home environments made up of two parents. With the exception of stress related to parenting, older mothers also appear to manage the emotional challenges of early parenthood better, in comparison to their teenage counterparts. They may have experienced less pre-existing psychological difficulties or have more resilience in coping with life's stressors.

In a prospective cohort study, McMahon et al (in press) noted that postnatal depression (PND) was not more prevalent in older mothers compared to those of any other age, but that women younger and older than 30 years of age may be at a greater risk of developing PND, thus indicating that the age of 30 is optimal for a successful postnatal adjustment in terms of depression. Whilst PND seems to occur at the usual prevalence rate for this group of mothers, anxiety appears to be increased, especially during pregnancy. This finding could be related to older mothers being made aware of their increased at risk status (Robb et al, 2005). For example, older mothers appear to be less attached to their developing fetus (Julia and Windridge, 1996) in early to mid-pregnancy, which could be explained by them experiencing fears of having a miscarriage or uncertainties resulting from antenatal screening for abnormalities (e.g. Loke and Poon, 2011). The recovery after childbirth and the physical demands of caring for a newborn baby may also explain anxieties in older mothers-to-be (e.g. Loke and Poon, 2011).

McMahon and colleagues (2011) examined the relationship between age, mode of conception and wellbeing in pregnancy in three groups of women of different ages who had conceived spontaneously (n = 295) and through assisted reproductive technologies (ART) (n = 297). In this study, older age was associated with lower levels of depression and anxiety, lower ratings of feeling controlled by their partner and greater psychological resilience, but also with lower levels of mother–fetus attachment. Maternal age was not related to feeling more anxious during pregnancy. However, having conceived through ART was associated with feeling more anxious but also with feeling more attached to the fetus, which seems to reflect that these women had more invested in their pregnancies emotionally. This study suggested that older first-time women have significant psychological advantages over their younger counterparts because they are better adjusted psychologically, and experience more support from their partners.

The negative influence of stress on parents, and mothers (as the main care provider) in particular, has been widely recognised. The impact of stress was examined in 82 primiparous women above the age of 35, at one and three months after delivery and again one year later. High levels of stress were noted at the one year follow-up. The degree of satisfaction expressed by mothers regarding their parenting role was linked to their confidence as well as their perceived support. One of the most significant mediators for parenting satisfaction was their relationship with their partner, who was a significant source of support for the mother. However, increased parenting stress cannot be assumed as a given phenomenon; some mothers and fathers did not report increased stress over this period of time. Indeed, couples who delayed parenthood were not substantially different to couples who become parents at a younger age (Garrison et al, 1997). It is important to note that the crucial element here was not the marital status or length of the relationship but the overall quality of the connection that the infant's parents had. Garrison and colleagues (1997), for example, stress that the quality of the relationship with the partner and other psychological factors are more important than age *per se* in predicting mood (both depression and anxiety) during pregnancy.

Overall, these findings strongly suggest that greater psychological resilience is related to good adjustment to motherhood. In addition, a range of advantageous sociodemographic factors associated with older mothers appears to enhance better adjustment to motherhood.

Transition to and experience of motherhood in older mothers

Older mothers may plan their pregnancies more carefully and this means they have certain expectations about motherhood, which can be realistic but which may also be unhelpful if they are not met. According to Dion (1995), unrealistic expectations have a negative impact on a woman's adjustment to motherhood and result in higher stress levels, partly because the woman may feel conflict, described as being 'torn apart' between being a career-oriented person and a child-focused mother. The feeling of being 'torn apart' (Clemmens, 2003) has also been expressed by teenage mothers and it is not an uncommon phenomenon for mothers who need to integrate the role of mother into their existing range of roles.

However, Dion's study (1995) of 114 women (aged 20–40 years) revealed that delayed childbearing was perceived to have certain advantages, some associated with personal development. The timing of the pregnancy was less related to expectations that parenthood would be fulfilling and more to family values and individual views of family functioning. Any delays in becoming a mother seemed to be because of educational and employment factors, especially if the mother's job required a sustained personal commitment, yet brought opportunities for self-expression and fulfilment. Whilst it seems that the pursuit of a career was important for some women, it was not the most important factor in determining pregnancy: the influence of the woman's peer group and the idea that parenthood could foster personal growth and wellbeing also played an important role in these women's reproductive decisions.

In a metasynthesis of the qualitative literature on women's reasons for delaying childbirth and their perceived 'at risk' status, Cooke and colleagues

(2010) suggest that women are faced with the issue of informed and uninformed decisions. Their analysis revealed that some women believed that they were better informed of risks than they actually were. These women were aware of some of the risks associated with delayed childbearing, such as the increased incidence of fetal abnormalities, but lacked information on other issues such as higher rates of late pregnancy complications. Other women had no knowledge of risks until they actually became pregnant. There was also a group of mothers who considered themselves to have been very well informed of the medical risks but still delayed childbearing. These findings highlight that older women appear to be influenced more by psychosocial factors than medical ones when they decide to become mothers.

Various studies have been undertaken exploring the transition to motherhood. For example, Berryman and Windridge (2007) examined the views and experiences of pregnancy and motherhood after the age of 40 in 100 primiparous and 246 multiparous women. Contrary to other studies, few mothers had delayed childbearing for career reasons. The authors also noted that first-time mothers differed from multiparae on a range of aspects, including family background, fertility problems and antenatal problems. Fertility issues were a major concern for first-time mothers, but in both groups a considerable number of babies were the result of unplanned pregnancies. Pregnancies were not perceived as being particularly problematic for these mothers, although many women experienced considerable anxiety regarding the possibility of having a baby with Down's syndrome, which may not be surprising given their age at conception. In a continuation of this project, Berryman and Windridge (1991b) explored how mothers aged 40 and over viewed parenthood, baby-feeding practices, and the baby–mother relationship. Expectations among primiparous and multiparous mothers varied in terms of the amount of tiredness, calmness and patience they believed they would experience, whilst both groups described similar breastfeeding practices. It is noteworthy that tiredness and lack of sleep did not seem to be overwhelming problems for mothers aged 40 and over.

According to one longitudinal study, which compared 54 older women (aged 35 and over) with 53 younger women (aged 20 to 29) as part of the Leicester Motherhood Project, healthcare professionals were more likely to place women over 35 in a 'high risk' category based on their age, but age *per se* did not present an obstetric risk factor (Windridge et al, 1999). Although older women believed that their infants were more vulnerable during labour and consequently they were more concerned and worried, they were also more positive towards the birth experience and less likely to blame staff for making their labour pain worse.

However, in Bornstein and colleagues' study (2006), older mothers reported more physical stress during labour and they recalled their babies as less well adjusted during the first month of their lives. Shelton and Johnson (2006) explored the narratives of older mothers, focusing on the dominant social ideals of the 'perfect mother' and the discrepancies between this ideal and reality. Their analysis revealed that mothers found it challenging and difficult to adapt to motherhood whilst integrating their different role and maternal identities. Their narratives were dominated by the cost of motherhood and the loss of personal freedom and associated lifestyle. A major theme in delayed parenthood described the loss of identity, youth, spontaneity, control, sanity, power, self-esteem, and connection with partner. Some of these factors were seen to contribute to the development of PND. Maternal ambivalence was very evident in their narratives, while the conflict between the idea of being a perfect mother and a good enough one was discussed at a wider societal level. Interestingly, an earlier study (Mercer 1986, cited in Reece, 1995) identified that older mothers experienced less gratification in parenting compared to younger mothers. Other studies have also noted that older mothers were more isolated, and felt conflict between career demands and motherhood, and hence experienced less positive attitudes towards mothering (Meisenhelder and Meservey, 1987).

Despite some of the concerns expressed by older mothers, they still seem to benefit from psychological and social advantages in their transition to motherhood, compared to teenage mothers. For example, according to Carolan's research (2005, 2006), older mothers take becoming a mother seriously, viewing it as a 'major life project' with clearly defined stages, which are marked by information gathering, extensive planning and preparation for the pregnancy, and preparing for the birth. Once the baby is born, older mothers realise that they need to adjust to caring for a dependant infant. This process was described in distinct stages: 'the nightmare of early mothering', the 'struggle and ambivalence' (i.e. feeling vulnerable and disempowered), the stage of 'giving in, realising, finding my own way', and, finally, by 'feeling like a mother' (Carolan, 2005: 769), which happens around 6–8 months after the birth. Although the process of adjustment as described here is comparable to that reported for teenage mothers and is not necessarily unique to mothers with an advanced maternal age, these two groups of mothers may differ in their psychological preparation for pregnancy and motherhood which may be a reflection of their economic and social backgrounds.

Nelson's (2004) qualitative study of older first-time mothers confirmed the view that older mothers actively prepare themselves for motherhood. Firstly, planned pregnancies are often the product of a long-held desire and, in the pursuit of motherhood, women educate themselves and remain positive even in the face of infertility issues. Secondly, older mothers are very clear as to what they want, partly because they have informed themselves about their options and decided on the ones best suited to them. According to Nelson (2004), 'they have been around' and they want to 'do this right'. In this context, the child is intensely appreciated and desired. Finally, older mothers have had time to consider and reorganise their priorities. They often perceive themselves as having a lot more to lose when having a child, but they also believe that they have a lot more to give. Interestingly, Nelson noted that older mothers actively seek to find advantages about delaying childbearing, while refusing to acknowledge potential medical risks (to self and baby) and disadvantages (such as fatigue, and the fact they may find themselves caring for their child as well as their aging parents).

Various studies comparing older and younger mothers highlight the better psychological adjustment of older women during pregnancy and throughout the first year of motherhood. In Robinson et al's (1988) comparison of 36 older first-time mothers (aged 35 years or older) with 31 younger women (aged 31 or less), both groups reported a reduction in marital intimacy but an increase in marital satisfaction. Compared to younger mothers, the older mothers seemed to have adopted a less traditional role and now demonstrated more autonomy in their personal styles. They were also more likely to have returned to full-time employment one year after the birth of their baby. A return to full-time employment may be a lifestyle choice as well as a desire to have a role other than being a full-time, stay-at-home mother.

The process of postnatal adjustment is not unique to older mothers and recurring themes are identifiable in the narratives of women of different ages. However, delayed childbearing may precipitate certain paradoxes such as the potential for the psychological benefits associated with older motherhood being outweighed by decreased capacity to meet the physical demands of caring for young children. It is not surprising that some older mothers have voiced concerns regarding their physical fitness. Dobrzykowski and Stern (2003) described this as feeling 'out of sync' which refers to the concepts of mortality (the clock ticking), vitality (physical fertility, plans for a second child, level of energy, etc.) and the larger society of which they are a member. However, the more confident a mother felt about her abilities to parent successfully, the less she felt socially pressured. Whilst older mothers may be concerned about their mortality and vitality, being older and more mature as a person with more life experience can be advantageous, too. Stark (1997) noted that younger gravidas had higher scores on fear of helplessness and loss of control during labour and birth, suggesting that life experience serves as a protective factor for older mothers. As older mothers are generally better educated, financially more secure, and seek prenatal care earlier, they may prepare for labour and birth differently by engaging more with services offering classes.

Interventions

As women who become pregnant after the age of 35 do not present with the same psychosocial disadvantages as teenage mothers, there is much less debate about possible social problems, and consequently, less emphasis has been placed on reducing pregnancy in mothers of this age group. For this reason, most interventions offered to these women fall into what other pregnant and postpartum mothers are routinely offered in healthcare settings. However, there are some issues that healthcare providers may like to consider when they are dealing with an older mother.

Nelson (2004) advises a three-pronged approach to intervening with older mothers:

- Anticipate their needs and concerns.
- Acknowledge and respect their knowledge and their desire for independence.
- Reassure them in their efforts.

Within this context, it is also important that healthcare professionals offer tailored or individualised antenatal as well as postnatal care, and that, throughout, the women's concerns, fears and expectations are acknowledged and normalised without being trivialised (Nelson, 2004).

An older woman's reasons for delaying motherhood should be explored in a non-judgemental manner and ultimately respected. Naturally, midwives and healthcare providers need to discuss medical risk factors with women but this communication should draw on the woman's desire for information without forcing the attention towards the risk itself (Cooke et al, 2010). Within a tailored healthcare approach for older women, a number of factors need to be explored and understood: their expectations about the pregnancy and life with a baby, the values that are placed on this particular pregnancy and its context (from being welcomed and wanted to the wider family environment) and their readiness and adaptation to becoming a mother (Suplee et al, 2007).

The need for ongoing social support with practical and emotional assistance may be less obvious to older mothers who may have been used to leading autonomous lives. However, they may feel isolated from other mothers because of their age, their socioeconomic standing and other sociodemographic factors. They may also find themselves having to look after an infant as well as aging parents. The degree of support they can expect from their partner may depend on the demands his job makes on him. Suplee and colleagues (2007) warn that, due to work demands, partners of professional women may be less available to provide support to new mothers and assist them to regain their psychological and physical strength in the immediate postpartum period. Hence, appropriate education about realistic expectations is important to facilitate a better adjustment in this group of women.

Older mothers may benefit from more advantageous starting points in their adjustment to motherhood alongside greater psychological maturity and resilience. However, the provision of appropriate guidance is an important aspect of individual or tailored healthcare for women of advanced maternal age. Whilst some of the above-mentioned psychological and social factors may place these women on a better trajectory for good maternal adjustment, it remains important to focus on providing reassurance and reviewing expectations, both during pregnancy and after, and assessing insecurities and vulnerability, isolation and sleep deprivation (Suplee et al, 2007).

Conclusions

Findings from studies exploring age in relation to motherhood suggest that women in different age groups may have varying experiences in relation to childbirth and parenting. However, maternal age alone may not be one of the strongest explanatory factors or predictors of long-term outcomes as its impact could be largely individual. A myriad of factors is shown to play a substantial role in the way a mother adjusts to being a mother and subsequently interacts with her infant. Most importantly, the parenting traditions, personal values and, above all, the preparedness and sense of right timing decide what each mother deems as important. Finally, the best mothers, and indeed parents, are the ones that are not defined by their age but rather by their interactions with their children, i.e. parents who are warm, loving and committed.

Discussion questions

- How are older mothers represented in the media?
- What type of parenting behaviours do older mothers tend to show?
- What personal and social characteristics does an older mother typically have?
- What impact does mood have on older mothers' parenting behaviours and attachment?
- What are the long-term outcomes for the infants of older mothers?
- What helps and hinders the transition to motherhood in older mothers?
- What interventions should be offered to older mothers?

References

Arensen J (1994) Strengths and self-perceptions of parenting in adolescent mothers. *Journal of Pediatric Nursing* **9**(4): 251–7

Aujoulat I, Libion F, Berrewaerts J, Noirhomme-Renard F, Deccache A (2010) Adolescent mothers' perspectives regarding their own psychosocial and health needs: A qualitative exploratory study in Belgium. *Patient Education and Counseling* **81**: 448–53

Barnet B, Liu JL, DeVoe M, Alperovitz-Bichell K, Duggan AK (2007) Home visiting for adolescent mothers: Effects on parenting, maternal life course, and primary care linkage. *Annals of Family Medicine* **5**(3): 224–32

Beers LA, Hollo RE (2009) Approaching the adolescent-headed family: A review of teen parenting. *Current Problems in Pediatric and Adolescent Health Care* **39**(2): 216–33

Belsky J (1999) Interactional and contextual determinants of attachment security. In J Cassidy and P Shaver (eds) *Handbook of attachment theory and research* (pp 249–64). New York: Guildford Press

Benzies K, Tough, S, Tofflemire K, Frick C, Faber A, Newburn-Cook C (2006) Factors influencing women's decisions about timing of motherhood. *Journal of Obstetric, Gynecologic and Neonatal Nursing* **35**: 625–33

Berlin LJ, Brandy-Smith C, Brooks-Gunn J (2002) Links between childbearing age and observed maternal behaviours with 14-month-olds in the early head start research and evaluation project. *Journal of Infant Mental Health* **23**(1–2): 104–29

Berryman JC, Windridge KC (1991a) Having a baby after 40: I. A preliminary investigation of women's experience of pregnancy *Journal of Reproductive and Infant Psychology* **9**: 3–18

Berryman JC, Windridge KC (1991b) Having a baby after 40: II. A preliminary investigation of women's experience of pregnancy *Journal of Reproductive and Infant*

Psychology **9**: 19–33

Berryman JC, Windridge KC (2007) Pregnancy after 35 and attachment to fetus. *Journal of Reproductive and Infant Psychology* **14**(2): 133–43

Bornstein MH, Putnick DL, Suwalsky JTD, Gini M (2006) Maternal chronological age, prenatal and perinatal history, social support, and parenting infants. *Child Development* **77**(4): 875–92

Breen AV, McLean KC (2010) Constructing resilience: Adolescent motherhood and the process of self-transformation. *Narrative Development in Adolescence* **20**(1): 151–68

Breheny M, Stephens C (2008) 'Breaking the cycle'. Constructing intergenerational explanations for disadvantage. *Journal of Health Psychology* **13**(6): 754–63

Brooks-Gunn J, Chase-Lansdale PL (1995) Adolescent parenthood. In: Bornstein MH (ed) *Handbook of parenting: Status and social conditions of parenting* (pp.113–49). Lawrence Erlbaum, Mahwah, NJ

Brooks-Gunn J, Furstenberg FF (1986) The children of adolescent mothers: Physical, academic, and psychological outcomes. *Developmental Review* **6**: 224–51

Brophy-Herb HE, Honig AS (1999) Reflectivity: Key ingredient in positive adolescent parenting. *Journal of Primary Prevention* **19**(3): 241–50

Campbell P (2011) Boundaries and risk: Media framing of assisted reproductive technologies and older mothers. *Social Science & Medicine* **72**: 265–72

Carolan M (2005) 'Doing it properly': The experience of first time mothering over 35 years. *Health Care for Women International* **26**(9): 764–87

Carolan M (2006) The project: Having a baby over 35. *Women and Birth* **20**: 121–6

Carolan M, Nelson S (2007) First mothering over 35 years: Questioning the association of maternal age and pregnancy risk. *Health Care for Women International* **28**: 534–55

Carter SL, Osofsky JD, Hann DM (1991) Speaking for the baby: A therapeutic intervention with adolescent mothers and their infants. *Journal of Infant Mental Health* **12**(4): 291–301

Clemmens D (2003) Adolescent motherhood: A meta-synthesis of qualitative studies. *American Journal of Maternal/Child Nursing* **28**(2): 93–9

Coley RL, Chase-Lansdale L (1998) Teenage pregnancy and parenthood: Recent evidence and future directions. *American Journal of Psychology* **53**: 152–66

Cooke A, Mills T, Lavender T (2010) "Informed and uninformed decision making": Women's reasoning, experiences and perceptions with regard to advanced maternal age and delayed childbearing: A meta-synthesis. *International Journal of Nursing Studies* **47**: 1317–29

Cooper PJ, Murray L (1998) Postpartum depression. *British Medical Journal* **316**: 1884–6

Cox J, Bevill L, Forsyth J, Missal S, Sherry M, Woods ER (2005) Youth preferences for prenatal and parenting teen services. *Journal of Pediatric and Adolescent Gynecology* **18**(3): 167–74

Cox JE, Buman M, Valenzuela J, et al (2008) Depression, parenting attributes and social support among adolescent mothers attending a teen tot program. *Journal of Pediatric and Adolescent Gynecology* **21**: 275–81

Crockenberg S (1986) Professional support for adolescent mothers: Who gives it, how adolescent mothers evaluate it. What they prefer. *Journal of Infant Mental Health* **7**(1): 49–58

Crockenberg S (1987) Predictors and correlates of anger toward and punitive control of toddlers by adolescent mothers and high risk infants' functioning in late infancy. *Child Development* **58**: 86–99

Deutscher B, Fewell RR, Cross M (2006) Enhancing the interactions of teenage mothers and their at-risk children: Effectiveness of a maternal-focused intervention. *Topics in Early Childhood Special Education* **26**(4): 194–205

Dion KK (1995) Delayed parenthood and women's expectations about the transition to parenthood. *Journal of Behavioral Development* **18**: 315–33

Dobrzykowski T, Stern P (2003) Out of sync: A generation of first time mothers over 30. *Health Care for Women International* **24**(3): 242–53

Dunst CJ, Vance SD, Cooper CS (1986) A social systems perspective of adolescent pregnancy determinants of parent and parent–child behaviour. *Journal of Infant Mental Health* **7**(1): 34–48

East PL, Felice ME (1990) Outcomes and parent–child relationships of former adolescent mothers and their 12-year-old children. *Journal of Developmental & Behavioral Pediatrics* **11**(4): 175–83

East PL, Matthews KL, Felice ME (1994) Qualities of adolescent mothers' parenting. *Journal of Adolescent Health* **15**: 163–8

Ensor R, Hughes C (2010) With a little help from my friends: Maternal social support, via parenting, promotes willingness to share in preschoolers born to young mothers. *Infant Child Development* **19**: 127–41

Faber NB (1991) The process of pregnancy resolution among adolescent mothers. *Adolescence* **26**: 697–716

Fergusson D, Woodward L (1999) Maternal age and educational and psychosocial outcomes in early adulthood. *Journal of Child Psychology and Psychiatry* **43**(3): 479–89

Figueireido B, Bifulco A, Pacheco A, Costa R, Magarinho R (2006) Teenage pregnancy, attachment style, and depression: A comparison of teenage and adult pregnant women in a Portuguese series. *Attachment & Human Development* **8**(2): 123–38

Flanagan PJ, McGrath MM, Meyer EC, Coll CT (1995) Adolescent development and transitions to motherhood. *Pediatrics* **96**: 273–7

Garrett SC, Tidwell R (1999) Differences between teenage mothers and nonmothers: An interview study. *Adolescence* **34**: 91–105

Garrison MEB, Blalock LB, Zarski JJ, Merritt PB (1997) Delayed parenthood: An exploratory study of family functioning. *Family Relations* **46**: 281–90

Grace JT (1989) Development of maternal–fetal attachment during pregnancy. *Nursing Research* **38**: 228–32

Hadfield L, Rudoe N, Sanderson-Mann J (2007) Motherhood, choice and the British media: A time to reflect. *Gender Education* **19**(2): 255–63

Harden A, Brunton G, Fletcher A, Oakley A (2009) Teenage pregnancy and social disadvantage: Systematic review integrating controlled trials and qualitative studies. *British Medical Journal* **339**: b4254

Harker L, Thorpe K (1992) "The last egg in the basket?" Elderly primiparity – a review of findings. *Birth* **19**(1): 23–9

Holub CK, Kershaw TS, Ethier KA, Lewis JB, Milan S, Ickovics JR (2007) Prenatal and parenting stress on adolescent maternal adjustment: Identifying a high risk subgroup. *Maternal and Child Health Journal* **11**: 153–9

Julia CB, Windridge KC (1996) Pregnancy after 35 and attachment to the fetus. *Journal of Reproductive and Infant Psychology* **14**(2):133–43

Kelly DM (1996) Stigma stories: Four discourses about teen mothers, welfare, and poverty. *Youth Society* **24**(7): 421

Keown LJ, Woodward LJ, Field J (2001) Language development of pre-school children born to teenage mothers. *Infant and Child Development* **10**: 129–45

Kumar R, Robson K (1984) A prospective study of emotional disorders in childbearing women. *British Journal of Psychiatry* **144**: 35–47

Lampinenen R, Vehvilaonen-Julkunen K, Kankkunen R (2009) A review of pregnancy in women over 35. *Open Nursing Journal* **3**: 33–8

Leadbeater BJ, Bishop SJ, Raver CC (1996) Quality of mother–toddler interactions, maternal depressive symptoms, and behavioral problems in preschoolers of adolescent mothers. *Developmental Psychology* **32**(2): 280–8

Letourneau NL, Stewart MJ, Barnfather AK (2004) Adolescent mothers: Support needs, resources, and support-education interventions. *Journal of Adolescent Health* **35**: 509–25

Loke AY, Poon CF (2011) The health concerns and behaviours of primigravida: Comparing advanced age pregnant women with their younger counterparts. *Journal of Clinical Nursing* **20**: 1141–50

Mayers HA, Hager-Bundy M, Buckner EB (2008) The chances for children teen parent–infant project: Results of a pilot intervention for teen mothers and their infants in inner city high schools. *Journal of Infant Mental Health* **29**(4): 320–42

Mayers HA, Siegler AL (2004) Finding each other: Using a psychoanalytic-developmental perspective to build understanding and strengthen attachment between teenage mothers and their babies. *Journal of Infant, Child and Adolescent Psychotherapy* **3**(4): 444–65

McMahon CA, Boivin J, Gibson FL, et al (2011) Age at first birth, mode of conception and psychological wellbeing in pregnancy: Findings from the parental age and transition to parenthood Australia (PAPTA) study. *Human Reproduction* **26**(6): 1389–98

McMahon CA, Boivin J, Gibson FL, et al (in press) Older first-time mothers and early postpartum depression: A prospective cohort study of women conceiving spontaneously or with assisted reproductive technologies. *Fertility and Sterility* (in press)

Meisenhelder JB, Meservey PM (1987) Childbearing over thirty: Description and satisfaction with mothering. *Western Journal of Nursing Research* **9**(4): 527–41

Miller BC, Benson B, Galbraith KA (2001) Family relationships and adolescent pregnancy risk: A research synthesis. *Developmental Reviews* **21**: 1–38

Mollborn S, Morningstar E (2009) Investigating the relationship between teenage childbearing and psychological distress using longitudinal evidence. *Journal of Health and Social Behavior* **50**(9): 310–26

Montgomery K (2002) Planned adolescent pregnancy: What they wanted. *Journal of Pediatric Health Care* **16**: 282–9

Nath PS, Barkowski JG, Whitman TL, Schellenbach CJ (1991) Understanding adolescent parenting: The dimensions and functions of social support. *Family Relations* **40**: 411–20

Nelson A (2004) A qualitative study of older first-time mothering in the first year. *Journal of Pediatric Health Care* **18**: 284–91

Nicolson P (1999) Loss, happiness and postpartum depression: The ultimate paradox. *Canadian Psychology* **40**(2): 162–78

Osofsky JJ, Hann DM, Peebles C (1993) Adolescent parenthood: Risks and opportunities for parents and infants. In: Zeanah CH (ed) *Handbook of infant mental health* (pp. 106–19). Guilford Press, New York

Osofsky JJ, Osofsky JD (1970) Adolescents as mothers. *American Journal of Orthopsychiatry* **40**: 825

Rafferty Y, Griffin KW, Lodise M (2011) Adolescent motherhood and developmental outcomes of children in early head start: The influence of maternal parenting behaviours, well-being, and risk factors within the family setting. *American Journal of Orthopsychiatry* **81**(2): 228–45

Ragozin AS, Basham RB, Crnic KA, Greenberg MT, Robinson NM (1982) Effects of maternal age on parenting role. *Developmental Psychology* **18**(4): 627–34

Reece S (1995) Stress and maternal adaptation in first-time mothers more than 35-years old. *Applied Nursing Research* **8**(2): 61–6

Reid V, Meadows-Oliver M (2007) Postpartum depression in adolescent mothers: An integrative review of the literature. *Journal of Pediatric Health Care* **21**(5): 289–98

Robb FV, Alder EM, Prescott RJ (2005) Do older primigravidas differ from youger primigravidas in their emotional experience of pregnancy? *Journal of Reproductive and Infant Psychology* **23**(2): 135–41

Robinson GE, Olmsted M, Garner DM, Gare DJ (1988) Transition to parenting in elderly primiparas. *Journal of Psychosomatic Obstetrics & Gynecology* **9**: 89–101

Samuels V, Stockdale D, Crase S (1994) Adolescent mothers' adjustment to parenting. *Journal of Adolescence* **17**: 427–43

Schmidt RM, Wiemann CM, Rickert VI, Smith B (2005) Moderate to severe depressive symptoms among adolescent mothers followed four years postpartum. *Journal of Adolescent Health* **38**: 712–18

Shaw M, Lawlor DA, Najman JM (2005) Teenage children of teenage mothers: Psychological, behavioral and health outcomes form Australian prospective longitudinal study. *Social Science & Medicine* **62**: 2526–39

Shaw R, Giles D (2009) Motherhood on ice? A media framing analysis of older mothers in the UK news. *Psychology and Health* **24**(2): 221–36

Shelton N, Johnson S (2006) I think motherhood for me was a bit like a double-edged sword: Narratives of older mothers. *Journal of Community and Applied Social Psychology* **16**: 316–30

Smith J, Bates PB (1999) Life-span perspectives on development. In MH Bornstein, ME Lamb (eds) *Developmental psychology: An advanced textbook* (4th edn, pp. 47–72). Erlbaum, Mahwah, NJ

Sommer K, Whitman T, Borkowski J, Schellenbach C, Mawell S, Keogh D (1993) Cognitive readiness and adolescent parenting. *Developmental Psychology* **18**: 627–34

Stark M (1997) Psychosocial adjustment during pregnancy: The experience of mature gravidas. *Journal of Obstetric, Gynecologic and Neonatal Nursing* **26**: 206–11

Suplee P, Dawley K, Bloch J (2007) Tailoring peripartum nursing care for women of advanced maternal age. *Journal of Obstetric, Gynecologic and Neonatal Nursing* **36**: 616–23

Turley RNL (2003) Are children of young mothers disadvantaged because of their mother's age or family background. *Child Development* **74**(2): 465–74

Unger D, Wandersman L (1988) The relations of family and partner support to adjustment of adolescent mothers. *Child Development* **59**: 1056–60

Viau PA (2002) An exploration of health concerns and health promotion behaviours in pregnant women over age 35. *American Journal of Maternal/Child Nursing* **27**(6): 328–34

Wayland J, Tate S (1993) Maternal–fetal attachment and perceived relationships with important others in adolescents. *Birth* **20**(4): 198–203

Wiemann CM, Rickert VI, Berenson, AB, Volk RJ (2005) Are pregnant adolescents stigmatized by pregnancy. *Journal of Adolescent Health* **325**: e.1–352.e7

Windridge K, Cert PG, Berryman JC (1999) Women's experiences of giving birth after 35. *Birth* **26**(1): 16–23

Chapter 7

Maternal age and mortality

Julie Maddocks

Introduction

This chapter examines the relationship between maternal age and mortality by presenting an outline of the background of the national confidential enquiries and the findings from the latest reports.

The focus is on the role of the enquiries in promoting learning from adverse events and how the findings can be used both to improve the health of mothers and babies, and to prevent morbidity and death. The impact of younger and older maternal age on mortality is discussed and key messages for health professionals are presented.

The national confidential enquiries

Until recently, there were three national confidential enquiries, the ultimate aims of which were to improve healthcare and reduce avoidable mortality:

- National Confidential Enquiry into Patient Outcome and Death (NCEPOD).
- Confidential Enquiry into Maternal and Child Health (CEMACH), later known as Centre for Maternal and Child Enquiries (CMACE).
- Confidential Inquiry into Suicide and Homicide by People with Mental Illness (CISH).

Confidential enquiries utilised a variety of methods including collection and analysis of epidemiological data, surveys, and panel enquiries. Dissemination of the findings and recommendations of the enquiries included printed and electronic reports, conferences, workshops, seminars, posters, and packages for cascading. Whatever approach was used, the identity of the patients, clinicians and healthcare providers was kept confidential, unless prior consent had been obtained for disclosure or there were reasonable grounds for believing that the enquiry had become aware of an illegal act or acts.

The origins of modern confidential enquires can be traced back to 1952, when the National Confidential Enquiries into Maternal Deaths (CEMD) was introduced in response to concerns over variable rates of avoidable maternal mortality in different parts of England. CEMD's remit was to assess the level, causes and contributors to maternal mortality and produce recommendations to address identified deficiencies in care. The enquiry utilises an observational approach, based on collating information on the deaths of women up to 12 months after the birth of their baby. Local coordinators, in all maternity units in England, Wales and Northern Ireland notify regional offices, using a standardised notification system. These data are entered into a database and the aggregated data are used to produce a three-year (triennial) maternal mortality report.

The value attached to Maternal Death Enquiry (MDE) findings by professionals over the past 50 years is reflected in the level of interest and attention generated by each new report. Although there is limited evidence for major impact of individual reports on changing practice (Hibbard and Milner, 1994), findings have had an important influence in certain areas. CEMD provided the impetus for national guidance on thromboprophylaxis for pregnant and postnatal women at risk of thromboembolism. More recently, the need to improve recognition of the deterioration and development of critical illness in pregnancy was highlighted, with recommendations leading to the widespread adoption of the modified obstetric early warning score in the UK (Lewis, 2007). The MDE has continued to receive support from those involved in national and strategic planning and policy of maternity services, including the Department of Health, the Royal College of Midwives and the Royal College of Obstetricians and Gynaecologists.

The Confidential Enquiry into Stillbirths and Deaths in Infants (CESDI) was established in 1992 by the Department of Health, with the aim of reducing late pregnancy losses, and deaths in the first few weeks of life, by identifying where suboptimal care might have contributed to a poor outcome (CESDI, 2003). CESDI covered deaths from the 20th week of pregnancy to the end of the first year of life, including late fetal losses and all stillbirths. A death was notified by a local co-ordinator to the regional office using a 'rapid report' notification form. This data enabled CESDI to provide accurate national data on the numbers and causes of stillbirth and infant death, which was reported in an annual report. CESDI also conducted detailed confidential enquiries into specific areas of concern, such as intrapartum stillbirth.

The Confidential Enquiries into Maternal and Child Health (CEMACH) was formed on 1st April 2003 by the amalgamation of the Confidential Enquiry into Stillbirths and Deaths in Infants (CESDI) and the Confidential Enquiry into Maternal Deaths (CEMD). In 2009 CEMACH changed its name to the Centre for Maternal and Child Enquiries (CMACE) and became a registered charity.

Centre for Maternal and Child Enquiries (CMACE)

CMACE's mission was to improve health outcomes for women, babies and children by undertaking confidential enquiries into maternal and child health, by disseminating findings and by making recommendations for practice. CMACE was an independent, non-profit-making body. The enquiry's contract with the principal funding body, the National Patient Safety Agency (NPSA) ended on the 31st March 2011. At the time of writing, no new contract has been awarded and currently there is no national maternal death enquiry or national perinatal surveillance in England.

As of the 1st September 2011, the Healthcare Quality Improvement Partnership (HQIP) became responsible for the management and commissioning of the clinical outcome review programmes, which encompass national confidential enquiries. June 2012 saw HQIP appoint MBRRACE-UK (Mothers and Babies - Reducing Risk through Audits and Confidential Enquiries across the UK) to run the national Maternal, Newborn and Infant Clinical Outcomes Review Programme with immediate effect.

MBRRACE-UK is a collaboration with members from the National Perinatal Epidemiology Unit (NPEU) at Oxford University; Leicester, Liverpool and Birmingham universities; University College London; Imperial College London; the stillbirth and neonatal death charity, Sands; and GP input (HQIP 2012).

Healthcare Quality Improvement Partnership (HQIP)

HQIP was established to promote quality in health and social care services in the UK, and in particular to increase the impact of clinical audit. It is led by a consortium including the Academy of Medical Royal Colleges and the Royal College of Nursing. HQIP is contracted by the Department of Health in England to deliver outcome-focused quality improvement programmes, structured around the collection of clinical data, including clinical audits, registers and confidential enquiries. HQIP is also tasked with promoting and developing other areas of quality improvement in health and social care. The objective of this work is to help assess the quality of healthcare and stimulate improvements in safety and effectiveness, by systematically enabling clinicians, managers and policy makers to learn from adverse events and other relevant data (Healthcare Quality Improvement Partnership, 2012).

Learning from adverse events

The confidential enquiry process requires assessment of anonymised case notes by local multidisciplinary regional panels of senior obstetricians, paediatricians, midwives, general practitioners, nurses, pathologists and others. Members are selected from different areas of the UK, to ensure that no individual would have had personal involvement with, or knowledge of, any of the cases. The direct involvement of clinicians has always been an important factor, as it ensures the relevance of findings for practice and support for the process amongst professionals.

National clinical audit

The Maternal Death Enquiry (MDE) is probably the oldest and longest-running clinical audit in the world. Clinical audit is recognised by the National Institute for Health and Clinical Excellence (NICE, 2002) as a quality improvement process that seeks to improve patient care and outcomes through systematic review of care against explicit criteria and the implementation of change. Aspects of the structure, processes, and outcomes of care are selected and systematically evaluated against explicit criteria. Where indicated, changes are implemented at an individual, team, or service level and further monitoring is used to confirm improvement in healthcare delivery. The MDE process reflects this cycle, in detailed assessment of individual cases, to learn lessons that can be applied generally. The quality of care is assessed with reference to predetermined standards, based on evidence, best practice and impact on outcomes. Evidence-based practice is fundamental to the provision of high quality, clinically effective, patient-centred care (Department of Health, 2000) and is achieved by evaluating ideas, practices and previous events and applying the learning achieved to current practice. The confidential enquiry reports contribute to evidence-based practice by the evaluation of what is known (outcome, i.e. maternal death) and done (care given, practice), and evaluating this against standards and best practice to decide what should influence what is done next (practice recommendations; *Figure 7.1*).

The General Medical Council (GMC) advises that all doctors must conduct regular audits. This medical and clinical data must be recorded honestly, and practice must be informed and improved based on the audit findings (General Medical Council, 2001). The UK Central Council for Nursing, Midwifery and Health Visiting stated that clinical governance, assisting the coordination of quality improvement initiatives such as clinical audit, is 'the business of every registered practitioner' (UK Central Council for Nursing, Midwifery and Health

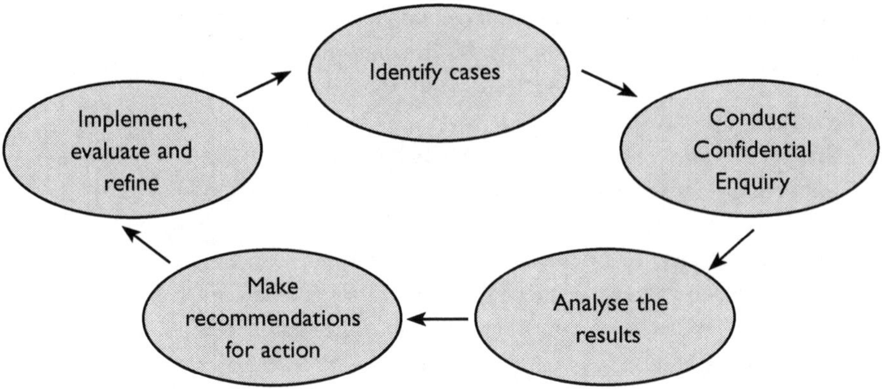

Figure 7.1 Audit cycle incorporating confidential enquiries. Source: CMACE, 2011.

Visiting, 2001). Senior doctors, midwives and nurses are key to the MDE process. They provide clinical leadership, which is an essential driver for development and refinement of effective working practices in all areas of the NHS. Clinical leaders are instrumental in addressing the quality aspects of service delivery, including guideline development, and setting and monitoring standards, all extremely important to ensure the clinical audit cycle is complete.

Maternal mortality

Mortality is defined as '…the condition of being mortal, or susceptible to death, the opposite of immortality' (Collins English Dictionary, 2011). The mortality rate is a measure of the number of deaths (in general, or due to a specific cause) in a specific population, scaled to the size of that population, per unit time. Mortality rate is typically expressed in units of deaths per 1000 individuals per year; thus, a mortality rate of 8.5 in a population of 100000 would mean 850 deaths per year in that entire population, or 0.85% out of the total. Mortality rate should be distinguished from morbidity rate, which refers to the number of individuals in poor health during a given time period (the prevalence rate) or the number of newly appearing cases of a disease per unit of time (incidence rate).

Maternal death

Maternal death is defined as: '... the death of a woman while pregnant or within 42 days of termination of pregnancy...from any cause related to the pregnancy or its management, but not from accidental or incidental causes' (World Health Organization, 2010: 4). Maternal deaths are classified as:

- Direct – obstetric causes.
- Indirect – existing conditions aggravated by pregnancy or its management.
- Incidental – unrelated to pregnancy.

It is a government requirement that all maternal deaths in the UK are subjected to confidential enquiry and consequently, all health professionals involved in the care of a woman who has died have a duty to provide the information required for the enquiry (Department of Health, 2001). The UK Maternal Death Enquiry, the oldest example of a maternal mortality and morbidity surveillance cycle, has now been internationally adopted by the World Health Organization (WHO) programme 'Beyond the numbers', which promotes the use of maternal death or morbidity reviews to make pregnancy safer around the world (World Health Organization, 2004).

CMACE produced the latest maternal mortality triennial report in March 2011 (CMACE, 2011b). In this triennium (2006–2008), 261 women in the UK died directly or indirectly as a result of pregnancy. The overall maternal mortality rate was 11.39 per 100 000 maternities. Direct deaths decreased from 6.24 per 100 000 maternities in 2003–2005 to 4.67 per 100 000 maternities in 2006–2008. The report highlighted a small decline in maternal mortality, the first in many years. This decrease was attributed, in part, to implementation of recommendations of previous enquiries which improved prevention and management of complications such as venous thromboembolism. The report also highlighted a reduction in social inequalities, with a significant decrease in maternal mortality in the most deprived areas of the UK and amongst women from the lowest socioeconomic groups. This could be attributed to the improvements in health services, which have extended access to and uptake of maternity services for vulnerable and socially excluded women. One of these innovations was 'Sure Start', an initiative that facilitated improved access by delivering maternity services in local venues such as Community Children Centres with flexible appointment times, including evenings and weekends (National Evaluation of Sure Start, 2008).

Older mothers and maternal mortality

The 2011 enquiry report (CMACE, 2011b) recognised the association between maternal age and risk of pregnancy-related death, confirming the findings of the previous triennial report, which highlighted that the highest maternal mortality

Table 7.1. The mean age for maternal deaths by major cause	
Cause	*Mean age*
Direct causes	
Thrombosis and thromboembolism	30
Pre-eclampsia	31
Haemorrhage	28
Amniotic fluid embolism	36
Sepsis	34
Indirect causes	
Cardiac disease	36
Deaths from psychiatric causes	30

rates were among the oldest women (Lewis, 2007). In *Saving mothers' lives* (CMACE, 2011b) the highest rates of maternal mortality were also recorded among older mothers; 95 of the 261 women who died were aged over 35 years, 24 were over 40 years, and the oldest was aged 47 years. Older mothers died from all major causes of death; however, there was a higher prevalence of cardiac-related deaths and amniotic fluid embolism (AFE). The report also highlighted for the first time a decline in the number of older mothers dying from thromboembolism (see *Table 7.1*).

Maternal death and cardiac disease

During the triennium 2006–2008, the most common cause of maternal death was cardiac disease. Fifty three women died from cardiac conditions associated with, or aggravated by, pregnancy. This equated to 2.31 per 100000 maternities representing an increase in the number and rate of maternal deaths from cardiac disease, a consistent trend over the last two triennial reports. The mothers who died from acquired heart disease ranged in age from 28 to 46 years, with a mean age of 36 years; three mothers were aged between 35 and 40 years and five mothers were over 40 years of age. Fifty one percent of the women who died from cardiac disease were deemed by assessors to have had some degree of substandard care.

The most important historic causes of cardiac-related maternal deaths, notably congenital heart disease and rheumatic heart disease, continue to decline. Deaths from sudden adult death syndrome, cardiomyopathy and particularly myocardial infarction have increased. This is likely to reflect a rising prevalence of risk factors for cardiovascular disease in the maternity population, particularly the increase in maternal obesity and the trend towards increasing age at childbirth. As these trends currently show no signs of reversal, the incidence of ischaemic heart disease and myocardial infarction during pregnancy is predicted to increase.

Key messages for health professionals

Ischaemic heart disease has now become a common cardiac cause of death in pregnancy and as such health professionals need to be aware of the associated risk factors (see *Box 7.1*).

Box 7.1. Risk factors associated with cardiac disease

- Obesity
- Age over 35 years
- Current smoker
- Pre-existing medical condition, such as diabetes or hypertension
- Family history of cardiac disease

Myocardial infarction in pregnancy can present with atypical features such as epigastric or abdominal pain, vomiting or dizziness. Midwives should maintain a low threshold for referral to an obstetrician or physician for further investigation. Women may not always be aware of the risks or take the necessary steps to seek medical advice. A pregnant woman with known cardiac disease must be referred for consultant-led care in a maternity service equipped with the appropriate expertise, including access to a cardiologist to care for the woman, which, in most cases, would be a tertiary level three unit.

Maternal death and amniotic fluid embolism (AFE)

AFE is an extremely rare obstetric complication but it carries a significant risk of maternal death. AFE occurs when amniotic fluid, fetal cells, fetal hair, or other debris from the fetus enter the mother's blood stream. Current theories suggest that this material triggers an allergic reaction, resulting in cardiorespiratory collapse and coagulopathy. AFE is one of the most common causes of maternal mortality in the world. In the triennium 2006–2008 in the UK, 13 women died of

AFE, they were aged 31–42 years, with a mean age of 36 years. The women who died in 2006–2008 were slightly older than in the previous triennial report where the median age was 33 years.

The UK-wide Obstetric Surveillance System (UKOSS) studies rare conditions in pregnancy. UKOSS differs from the MDE as it collects information on all confirmed or suspected cases, not just those where the woman died. In 2011, the UKOSS morbidity study found no association of AFE with increased age in the overall study population. However, an association with increased age was identified in women from ethnic minorities. The UKOSS data demonstrated that AFE was significantly associated with induction of labour and multiple pregnancy. There was also an association between caesarean delivery and postnatal amniotic fluid embolism (Knight et al, 2010).

The clinical presentation of AFE can be confusing and is still not completely understood (Tuffnell, 2003) but effective resuscitation is an essential response, irrespective of the underlying cause of collapse. Good outcomes are dependent on the place of maternal collapse and effective resuscitation (see *Box 7.2*).

Box 7.2. Risks factors associated with AFE

- Induction of labour
- Multiple pregnancy
- Caesarean birth

Maternal death and thromboembolism

There was a significant fall in the number of maternal deaths attributed to thrombosis and/or thromboembolism and no deaths of women over 40 years of age from thromboembolism in 2006–2008 (CMACE, 2011b). Prior to 1997, there was a sharp increase in risk of thrombosis for mothers over 40 years of age. The reduction in the numbers of deaths has been attributed to the introduction of national guidelines for thromboprophylaxis and better recognition of risk factors. There were four deaths of mothers aged between 35 and 39 years of age. These women were all overweight (body mass index 25–30) or obese (body mass index ≥35).

CMACE conducted a national three-year obesity and pregnancy project in 2010. As part of this project, extensive prospective data were collected from a cohort of 5068 women with maternal obesity (body mass index ≥35), who gave

Box 7.3. Risk factors associated with thromboembolism

- Age over 35 years of age
- Obesity
- Positive family history of thrombosis and/or thromboembolism
- Long periods of immobility

birth in the UK during March and April, 2009. The report concluded that maternal age over 35 years is a predictive factor for maternal obesity. Maternal age less than 20 years and over 35 years was a risk factor for poor pregnancy outcomes among severely obese women (CMACE, 2010).

The key messages for health professionals in relation to risk factors for thromboembolism are outlined in *Box 7.3*.

Risk assessment in early pregnancy continues to be the key factor in reducing mortality. Obesity remains the most important risk factor; the national obesity guidelines (CMACE/RCOG, 2010) should be implemented and audited by NHS trusts.

Young mothers and mortality

Thirteen mothers under the age of 20 died in the period 2006–2008; the youngest was aged 15 and four were aged between 15 and 16 (CMACE, 2011b). Seven of the 13 young mothers were known to social services; two were living in the care of social services and one was deemed homeless having recently been discharged from the care of social services. Two of the younger women were described as being 'learning disabled' and two used illegal drugs. No single cause of maternal death was associated with young maternal age, but there was an increased prevalence of stillbirth among younger mothers compared to mothers aged 25–29 (CMACE, 2011a).

Despite the widespread availability of guidance, a common theme through the enquiries was the lack of appropriate risk assessment and/or actions following identification of risk factors, especially complex social risk factors. Local clinical policies should be readily accessible at all times and reflect the most recent national guidance for the safe management of pregnant women and newborn babies.

The antenatal booking assessment is the most important assessment during pregnancy. The skills and clinical acumen of the midwife (and of other professionals involved) are essential to make a thorough assessment and act appropriately on the findings. With the introduction of the 2008 NICE antenatal guidelines and the use of standardised maternity records this task has been simplified, with prompts and evidence-based guidance available and accessible to all midwives and other healthcare professionals.

Case study

Mary was in her late 30s. She had four children aged between 2 and 10 years. At the time of booking her BMI was 35, she smoked at least 20 cigarettes per day, she had suffered from asthma and hypertension and had a family history of heart disease.

Mary booked at 13 weeks' gestation and was seen predominantly by her community midwife and GP who was monitoring her blood pressure. During a routine antenatal assessment at 36 weeks by her midwife, she complained of intermittent mild chest pain, shortness of breath, dizziness and vomiting. She was advised to see her GP. She did not make an appointment with her GP. She was found dead at her home one week later. A post mortem examination found coronary atheroma and the cause of death was myocardial infarction.

Discussion question

- How should Mary's care have been different and would this have prevented her death?

Author's comments

Mary had several risk factors for cardiac disease, which were highlighted at the point of entry to maternity care; therefore she should have been referred for consultant-led care. Although the midwife did refer to the GP when she complained of mild chest pain, given her history she should have been referred directly to hospital where a full assessment might have changed the outcome. Mary had had previous pregnancies and had her blood pressure routinely checked by her GP; she may have been reassured by seeing the midwife and unaware of her increased risk of heart attack as her pregnancy progressed. There was no documented evidence that the woman was informed of her risk factors nor any documented evidence of any discussions related to her high-risk status.

Conclusion

Maternal deaths are rare in the UK and it is reassuring that the mortality rate has declined in the last triennial report. Most health professionals recognise their duty to learn from every tragic event. The evidence from the Maternal Death Enquiry reports demonstrates that being a younger or older mother can increase the likelihood of this rare event and that there is scope to improve the recognition of risk factors and management of high risk women to reduce mortality and morbidity even further.

References

Centre for Maternal and Child Enquiries (2010) *Maternal obesity in the UK. Findings from a national project.* CMACE, London

Centre for Maternal and Child Enquiries (2011a) *Perinatal mortality 2009: United Kingdom.* CMACE, London

Centre for Maternal and Child Enquiries (2011b) Saving mothers' lives: Reviewing maternal deaths to make motherhood safer: 2006–08. The Eighth Report on Confidential Enquiries into Maternal Deaths in the United Kingdom. *British Journal of Obstetrics and Gynaecology* **118**(Suppl. 1): 1–203

Centre for Maternal and Child Health, Royal College of Obstetricians and Gynaecologists (2010) *Management of women with obesity in pregnancy.* CMACE/RCOG, London

Confidential Enquiry into Stillbirths and Deaths in Infancy (2003) *Eigth Annual Report.* The Stationery Office, London

Collins English Dictionary (2011) Available from: http://www.collinsdictionary.com

Department of Health (2000) *The NHS plan: A plan for investment, a plan for reform.* HMSO, London

Department of Health (2001) *Building a safer NHS for patients.* HMSO, London

General Medical Council (2001) *Good medical practice* (3rd edn). GMC, London

Healthcare Quality Improvement Partnership (2012) Available from: http://www.hqip.org.uk/

Hibbard B, Milner D (1994) Reports on confidential enquiries into maternal deaths: An audit of previous recommendations. *Health Trends* **26**(1): 26–8

Knight M, Tuffnell D, Brocklehurst P, Spark P, Kurinczuk JJ, UK Obstetric Surveillance System (2010) Incidence and risk factors for amniotic-fluid embolism. *Obstetrics and Gynecology* **115**(5): 910–7

Lewis G (ed) (2007) *Saving mothers' lives: Reviewing maternal deaths to make motherhood safer: 2003–05. The Seventh Report on Confidential Enquiries into Maternal Deaths in the United Kingdom.* CEMACH, London

National Advisory Body for Confidential Enquiry into Stillbirths and Deaths in Infancy

(1996) *Third annual report.* Department of Health, London

National Evaluation of Sure Start (2008) *The impact of Sure Start local programmes on three year olds and their families*. Available from: http://www.ness.bbk.ac.uk/impact/documents/42.pdf

National Institute for Health and Clinical Excellence (2002) *Principles for best practice in clinical audit*. Radcliffe Medical Press, Oxford

National Institute for Health and Clinical Excellence (2008) *Antenatal care, routine care for healthy pregnant women. Clinical guideline 62*. Available from: www.nice.org.uk/CG062

Tuffnell DJ (2003) Amniotic fluid embolism. *Current Opinion in Obstetrics and Gynaecology* **15**: 119–22

UK Central Council for Nursing, Midwifery and Health Visiting (2001) *Professional Self-regulation and clinical governance*. United Kingdom Central Council for Nursing, Midwifery and Health Visiting, London

World Health Organization (2004) *Beyond the Numbers – Reviewing maternal deaths and complications to make pregnancy safer*. WHO, Geneva. Available from: www.who.int/reproductive-health

World Health Organization (2010) *ICD 10 International statistical classification of diseases and related health conditions. 10th revision.* WHO, Geneva. Available from: http://apps.who.int/classifications/icd10/browse/2010/en

Index

I

L

M

N

O

P

R

S